American Pharmacists Association
BASIC PHARMACY & PHARMACOLOGY SERIES

Medication Workbook
for Pharmacy Technicians
A PHARMACOLOGY PRIMER

David R. Bright

Raabe College of Pharmacy
Ohio Northern University

Mary F. Powers

College of Pharmacy and Pharmaceutical Sciences
University of Toledo

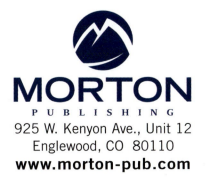

MORTON
PUBLISHING
925 W. Kenyon Ave., Unit 12
Englewood, CO 80110
www.morton-pub.com

Book Team

Publisher	Douglas Morton
Editor/Project Manager	Dona Mendoza
Production	Joanne Saliger
Interior/Cover Design	Bob Schram, Bookends

To the best of the Publisher's knowledge, the information presented in this book is correct and compatible with standards generally accepted for administering drugs. The reader is advised to consult the information material included with each drug or agent before administration. However, please note that you are responsible for following your employer's and your state's policies, procedures, and guidelines.

The job description for pharmacy technicians varies by institution and state. Your employer and state can provide you with the most recent regulations, guidelines, and practices that apply to your work.

The Publisher of this book disclaims any responsibility whatsoever for any injuries, damages, or other conditions that result from your practice of the skills described in this book for any reason.

ISBN 13: 978-0-89582-883-5

Library of congress Control Number: 2010931986

Printed in the United States of America

10 9 8 7 6 5 4 3 2 1

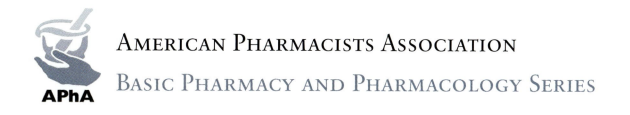

AMERICAN PHARMACISTS ASSOCIATION
BASIC PHARMACY AND PHARMACOLOGY SERIES

Dear Student or Instructor,

The American Pharmacists Association (APhA), the national professional society of pharmacists, and Morton Publishing Company, a publisher of educational texts and training materials in health care, are pleased to present this outstanding textbook, *Medication Workbook for Pharmacy Technicians: A Pharmacology Primer.* It is one of a series of distinctive texts and training materials in basic pharmacy and pharmacology published under this banner: American Pharmacists Association Basic Pharmacy and Pharmacology Series.

Each book in the series is oriented toward developing an understanding of fundamental concepts. In addition, each presents applied and practical information on the skills necessary to function effectively in positions below the prescriber level, such as pharmacy technicians and medical assistants, that involve working with medications. The role of such occupations in health care is increasingly important. The books in the series feature a visual design to enhance understanding and ease of use and are accompanied by various instructional support materials. We think you will find them to be valuable training tools.

The American Pharmacists Association and Morton Publishing thank you for using this book and invite you to look at other titles in this series, which are listed below.

Thomas E. Menighan, BPharm, MBA, ScD
Executive Vice President
Chief Executive Officer
American Pharmacists Association

Douglas N. Morton
President
Morton Publishing Company

TITLES IN THIS SERIES:
The Pharmacy Technician, Fourth Edition
The Pharmacy Technician Workbook and Certification Review, Fourth Edition
Medication Workbook for Pharmacy Technicians: A Pharmacology Primer

About the Authors

David R. Bright, Pharm.D., R.Ph., is Assistant Professor of Pharmacy Practice at the Raabe College of Pharmacy, Ohio Northern University, in Ada, Ohio. He received his bachelor of science in pharmaceutical sciences and doctor of pharmacy degrees from the University of Toledo and has also completed a Community Pharmacy Residency.

Mary F. Powers, Ph.D., R.Ph., is Professor of Pharmacy Practice at the College of Pharmacy and Pharmaceutical Sciences, University of Toledo, in Toledo, Ohio. She received her pharmacy degree from the University of Toledo and her doctor of philosophy in medical sciences degree from the Medical College of Ohio. Powers has extensive experience is community pharmacy practice and has also served as the Pharmacy Technician Program Coordinator at Mercy College of Northwest Ohio. She has been involved in teaching pharmacy technicians since 1998.

Artwork and Photography Credits

Morton Publishing, Inc., is thanked for generously providing the artwork from their titles *Exploring Anatomy & Physiology in the Laboratory* and *Case Mysteries in Pathophysiology*. The artwork enhances most of the chapters in the book so that students can have a visual image of the tissues and organs that are affected by medications.

Additionally, photographs of medications have been graciously provided by their manufacturers and can be found throughout the book. We thank the following companies for providing photographs of their medications: American Regents, Inc.; A Luitpold Pharmaceuticals, Inc. Company; Hospira Inc.; Eli Lilly and company; and Pfizer Inc.

Preface

This book is intended as a study aid for pharmacy technicians to build a functional foundation of knowledge about medications to work in a pharmacy and to prepare for the certified pharmacy technician exam. As the title implies, *Medication Workbook for Pharmacy Technicians: A Pharmacology Primer* is an introductory text for pharmacology and can serve to prepare the student for more challenging pharmacology textbooks. It can also be used as a companion to other textbooks. Although we initially developed the book for pharmacy technician training programs, it will also be useful for pharmacy technicians working in the field, as well as students in other health care professions who are studying pharmacology for the first time.

Pharmacology is a complex subject, and learning about medications can be challenging. The authors recommend that users of the workbook make flash cards to help memorize key points. In learning the generic names of medications, it may be helpful to focus on United States Adopted Names stems. Mastery of the material can also be enhanced by studying in groups and reviewing the material with other students or colleagues.

Workbook for Pharmacy Technicians: A Pharmacology Primer is divided into 15 chapters, followed by six appendices.

℞ The first three chapters of the book provide a basic introduction to the practice of pharmacy and the use of medications

℞ The remaining 12 chapters are devoted to providing the following:

- a basic description of anatomy and physiology,
- a primer on pharmacology actions,
- sample prescriptions,
- a list of USAN stems to help identify general categories of medications, and
- a brief overview of alternative therapies for several classes of medications.

℞ The chapters are concisely and clearly written with foundational information about the topics in each chapter, along with tables so that the student can readily find and remember information.

℞ Learning Objectives and Key Terms can be found at the beginning of each chapter.

℞ Each chapter ends with a summary, along with practice problems to help the technician study and learn the material.

℞ The appendices provide selected answers to practice problems as well as listings of

- Top 200 brand medications
- Top 200 generic medications
- Top 100 over-the-counter and health and beauty care products

- Top 100 hospital medications
- Common medications requiring refrigeration
- Institute for Safe Medication Practice's (ISMP) List of Error-Prone Abbreviations, Symbols, and Dose Designations

Additionally, password-protected Instructor Ancillaries are available online. The ancillaries include:

- Sample course outlines for 6-week, 10-week, and 15-week courses
- PowerPoint Presentation files containing information from the introduction of each chapter as well as ten sample multiple choice quiz questions.
- Sample prescriptions (as PowerPoint slides) that can be used as in-class quizzes or teaching tools for prescription interpretation that apply to each chapter
- A comprehensive exam (90-item) at the end of the instructor's manual

Acknowledgments

The authors thank Verender Gail Brown, B.S., R.Ph.T., C.Ph.T., Pharmacy Technician Educator at Anthem College—Orlando and member of the APhA Books and Electronics Products Editorial Advisory Board, for providing a detailed review of the book, along with several good suggestions for improvements. We also thank Julian I. Graubart, Senior Director, Books and Electronic Products, at APhA for his work toward co-branding the book with Morton Publishing. We are also grateful to Rebecca Schonscheck C.Ph.T., B.S., Director of Curriculum Development, Anthem Education Group, Phoenix, Arizona, and Bobbi Steelman, C.Ph.T., PTCB and ICPT, Daymar Institute, Bowling Green, Kentucky, Pharmacy Technician Program Manager, for providing reviews and helpful suggestions.

Finally, thank you to our supporting colleagues, family, and friends, including but certainly not limited to Judith A. Jones, Ph.D., and Heather and Lainey Bright.

Sincerely,
David R. Bright and Mary F. Powers

Contents

CHAPTER ONE

Introduction to Common Medications

1

KEY TERMS

Anatomy

Arthritis

Brand name

Cardiovascular

Complementary and alternative medicine (CAM)

Dermatologic

Diabetes

Drugs

Evidence-based medicine

Gastrointestinal

Generic name

Gross anatomy

Hematology

Microscopic anatomy

Oncology

Pathophysiology

Pharmacology

Physiology

Pneumonia

Receptors

Respiratory

Skeletal

United States Adopted Names (USAN) Council

LEARNING OBJECTIVES

After completing this chapter, the student will be able to:

1. Define the term *medication*
2. Describe why medications are prescribed
3. List 12 classifications for medications based on therapeutic use
4. Describe how drugs are named
5. Define USAN stems
6. Identify three nonmedicinal therapies
7. Define the terms *anatomy, physiology,* and *pathophysiology*
8. Explain the relationships among the pharmacy, the pharmacist, and the pharmacy technician
9. List 10 tasks that are commonly performed by pharmacy technicians
10. Describe the medication dispensing process and the role of the pharmacy technician in that process

What is a Medication? Why Do We Use Medications?

Advances in medicine and medical care, including developments with new medications, are among the changes in society that have contributed to people living longer and healthier lives in the past century.

Medications or **drugs** can be thought of as chemical substances that help people, as well as animals, maintain healthy living. Drugs have been defined as substances intended for use in the diagnosis, cure, mitigation, treatment, or prevention of disease in humans or other animals, as well as articles (other than food) intended to affect the structure or any function of the body of humans or other animals. Accepted uses for medications are based on substantial scientific testing that produces evidence of the effectiveness of a medication. Prescribing medications for clinical use on the basis of scientific data is termed **evidence-based medicine**.

Knowing the following terms will be helpful as you learn about the practice of pharmacy, the role of the pharmacy technicians, and the types of medications that are commonly dispensed in pharmacies:

Anatomy: the scientific study of the structure of living things

Arthritis: a condition associated with inflammation and damage to the joints of the body

Brand name: a unique, proprietary name selected by the pharmaceutical company that produces a drug

Cardiovascular: a term relating to the heart and blood vessels

Complementary and alternative medicine (CAM): therapies outside of evidence-based medicine

Dermatologic: referring to skin, hair, and nails

Diabetes: a chronic condition associated with how the body processes sugar that can be life-threatening

Drugs: substances intended for use in the diagnosis, cure, mitigation, treatment, or prevention of disease

Evidence-based medicine: prescribing medications for clinical use on the basis of scientific data

Gastrointestinal: referring to digestive activities (e.g., stomach, intestines)

Generic name: a specific, nonproprietary name assigned to a drug by the United States Adopted Names (USAN) Council

Gross anatomy: the study of structures within the body that are large enough to be seen by the naked eye

Hematology: study of the blood

Microscopic anatomy: the study of structures within the body that can be seen only with microscopes

Oncology: the study of cancerous diseases

Pathophysiology: the study of abnormal body functions that can be caused by diseases or other processes that are not normal

Pharmacology: the study of how drugs or other chemicals work in the body

Physiology: the study of the functions within living things

Pneumonia: one type of lung infection that can be treated with anti-infective medications

Receptors: minute specialized surfaces that provide the sites of actions for medications in different parts of the body

Respiratory: referring to lungs and other breathing passages

Skeletal: referring to bones

United States Adopted Names (USAN) Council: the group sponsored by the American Medical Association (AMA), United States Pharmacopeial Convention (USPC), and the American Pharmacists Association (APhA) that assigns generic names to drugs; the council determines generic names for drugs using special syllables called "stems," which can then be grouped by therapeutic class or category

There are many types of medications with many uses. The science of medications, including their chemical makeup, how they are processed in the body, how they are used to treat diseases and conditions, and the dangers associated with their use is termed *pharmacology*. In the study of pharmacology, there are several ways to classify medications, such as grouping by chemistry or by therapeutic uses. Chapter 3 provides an introduction to basic pharmacology.

In this book, medications are classified by their therapeutic uses in the following categories:

Anti-infective medications are taken to treat sickness caused by infections. Illnesses of this nature were life-threatening before the widespread use of anti-infective medications to treat diseases such as pneumonia.

Cardiovascular medications are taken for many reasons associated with diseases of the heart and blood vessels. High blood pressure and high blood cholesterol, along with many diseases of the heart, can be controlled with cardiovascular medications.

Diabetes is a chronic condition of the endocrine system associated with how the body processes sugar; this disorder can be life-threatening. Significant medical advances in the past century have allowed people with diabetes to live better lives. Like diabetes, thyroid conditions are also disorders of the endocrine system. The thyroid gland is an important organ in the body and provides important hormones that regulate a variety of body processes. **Thyroid** conditions can also be treated with prescription medications.

Diseases and conditions affecting the **bones** and **joints** as well as the **muscles** can be painful and debilitating. Arthritis is one example of a condition associated with damage to the joints of the body. Medications prescribed to treat arthritis have improved the quality of life and mobility of people afflicted with the disease. Medications with effects on the muscles in the body range from muscle relaxants to drugs that are used to treat chronic conditions such as muscular dystrophy. Muscular and skeletal medications have been helpful for people with muscular injuries or diseases to gain functional mobility.

In the past 50 years, many medications have been developed with effects on the **nervous system.** Disorders and conditions of the nervous system are many and range from attention deficit hyperactivity disorder (ADHD) to Alzheimer's disease to seizure disorders such as epilepsy. More common conditions such as anxiety and depression can also be treated with medications that affect the nervous system.

Respiratory medications are used to treat conditions of the lungs and other breathing passages. Conditions treated with respiratory medications range from common symptoms associated with coughs, colds, or allergies, as well as chronic diseases such as asthma.

Gastrointestinal medications are used to treat conditions associated with the digestive activities in the body. Commonly treated conditions range from constipation to diarrhea, gastroesophageal reflux, heartburn and indigestion, nausea, and vomiting. This category can also include medications used to treat obesity.

Reproductive medications can be associated with hormone therapy and also include nonhormonal medications that enhance the performance of reproductive organs. **Urinary medications** are drugs that affect urination and most commonly are prescribed to relieve urinary difficulties and treat urinary incontinence or painful urination.

Medications to treat conditions of the **eyes, ears, nose, mouth, and throat** are sometimes grouped together. Some of the most common conditions of the eye that are treated with medications are infections, glaucoma, and allergies. Some of the most common conditions of the ear that are treated with medications are infections, pain, and earwax buildup. Most of the conditions affecting the nose have effects throughout the respiratory system, as do medications used to treat conditions of the nose. Medications that treat conditions of the mouth and throat are most commonly associated with dental hygiene and sore throat.

Dermatologic medications are those used to treat conditions of the skin, hair, and nails. Dermatologic

conditions can include athlete's foot, dandruff, and nail fungus.

Hematology medications are drugs that affect the blood and can range from medications that affect bleeding as well as the components of the blood. **Oncology medications** are drugs used to treat different types of cancers. Hematology and oncology are two specialty areas of medicine that are often grouped together.

How Are New Drugs Named?

When new drugs reach the market, they have both a generic name and a brand name. Generic names, or nonproprietary names, are determined by the United States Adopted Names (USAN) Council, while the brand names, or proprietary names, are determined by their manufacturers. Brand names are also known as trade names.

The USAN Council is sponsored by the American Medical Association (AMA), United States Pharmacopeial Convention (USPC), and the American Pharmacists Association (APhA). Generic names provide some indication of the therapeutic or chemical class of the drug and should be unlikely to be confused with other drug names. The names for generic drugs involve using standardized syllables known as stems, which are put together to form the generic name. The USAN has a recommended list of stems, which is updated regularly (see http://www.ama-assn.org/ama1/pub/upload/mm/365/stem-list-cumulative.pdf). Examples of stems are provided in Table 1-1.

Examples of USAN stems are featured throughout this workbook in sections called **"What's in a name?"**

Additional Nonmedicinal Therapies

Medications can be thought of as specific and specialized chemicals that can be taken to treat or prevent diseases or conditions. Other nonmedicinal therapies

Table 1-1. Examples of USAN Stems

Stem	Description	Example
-caine	Local anesthetics	Lidocaine
-cort-	Cortisone derivatives	Hydrocortisone
-cycline	Tetracycline-derivative antibiotics	Minocycline
-olol	Propranolol-type beta-blockers	Atenolol
-pril	Angiotensin converting enzyme inhibitor-type antihypertensives	Enalapril

can also have beneficial effects. The term *complementary and alternative medicine* (CAM) includes therapies outside of evidence-based medicine. Often, CAM therapies are not as rigorously tested for safety and efficacy compared with evidence-based medicine therapies. Examples of CAM include prayer, herbs, nutritional supplements, meditation, chiropractic, yoga, diet, and exercise.

Besides CAM, other nonmedicinal therapies can be useful and important to treat diseases and conditions. Some examples are counseling, physical therapy, and the use of assistive devices.

The Science of Medications

Medications produce their effects because of interactions that occur at the submicroscopic level. Minute specialized surfaces called receptors provide the sites of actions for medications in different parts of the body.

To gain insight into how and why drugs work, it is important to learn basic information about anatomy and physiology. Anatomy can be thought of as the scientific study of the structure of living things. The study of anatomy is commonly divided into two parts: gross anatomy and microscopic anatomy. Gross anatomy can be thought of as the study of structures within the body that are large enough that they can be seen with the naked eye. Microscopic anatomy studies smaller structures within the body that can be seen with microscopes. Physiology can be thought of as the study of the functions within living things. The study of physiology gives us information about how different parts of the body work. Pathophysiology is a branch of physiology that studies abnormal body functions that can be caused by disease or other abnormal processes.

Medications and Pharmacies

Pharmacies are the places where medications are dispensed by pharmacists. Pharmacies can be found in a variety of places, including hospitals, grocery stores, mass merchandise stores, mail-order businesses, and traditional drugstores.

The **pharmacist** is the health care professional who practices the science of pharmacy. Pharmacists have knowledge and experience to help ensure the safe and effective use of medications. Pharmacists are required to have licenses to practice pharmacy, and the licenses are issued by state governmental agencies. One of the main activities performed by pharmacists is the safe and accurate dispensing of prescription medications. Pharmacists also commonly perform other activities associated with safe and effective

medication use, including medication counseling, providing information about drugs and their uses, and reviewing drug utilization (Figure 1-1).

Pharmacy technicians are support staff who work under the direct supervision of licensed pharmacists. Pharmacy technicians can assist pharmacists by performing routine tasks associated with preparing prescriptions for patients. Technicians are often required to meet standard competency in the field by obtaining certification.

Some common tasks performed by technicians include the following:

- ℞ Entering data into computers
- ℞ Counting tablets and capsules
- ℞ Placing medications in prescription bottles
- ℞ Billing insurance companies for goods and services
- ℞ Resolving billing and insurance problems
- ℞ Managing inventory
- ℞ Answering telephones
- ℞ Sending and receiving faxes
- ℞ Interacting with patients
- ℞ Operating cash registers
- ℞ Operating automated dispensing systems
- ℞ Complying with quality assurance practices
- ℞ Communicating via e-mail
- ℞ Maintaining and organizing necessary records
- ℞ Assisting with preparation of reports
- ℞ Scheduling consultation appointments
- ℞ Processing invoices and bills

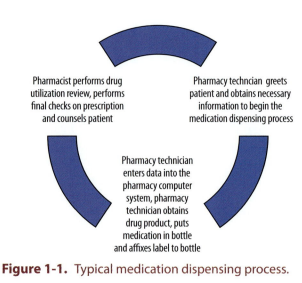

Pharmacist performs drug utilization review, performs final checks on prescription and counsels patient

Pharmacy techncian greets patient and obtains necessary information to begin the medication dispensing process

Pharmacy technician enters data into the pharmacy computer system, pharmacy technician obtains drug product, puts medication in bottle and affixes label to bottle

Figure 1-1. Typical medication dispensing process.

Chapter Summary !

Today, people live longer and healthier lives than ever before, in part due to advances with medications. Nonmedicinal therapies can also be helpful in the treatment and prevention of disease. Pharmacies are places where people go to get medications, and pharmacists dispense the medications. Pharmacy technicians play an important role in assisting pharmacists.

STUDENT NAME _____

DATE _____ INSTRUCTOR'S NAME _____

Match the following abbreviation with its meaning:

1. _____ Anatomy

2. _____ Arthritis

3. _____ Cardiovascular

4. _____ Complementary and alternative medicine (CAM)

5. _____ Dermatologic

6. _____ Diabetes

7. _____ Drugs

A. a term related to the heart and blood vessels

B. therapies outside of evidence-based medicine

C. a condition associated with damage to the joints of the body

D. the scientific study of the structure of living things

E. referring to skin, hair, and nails

F. articles intended for use in the diagnosis, cure, mitigation, treatment, or prevention of disease

G. a chronic condition associated with how the body processes sugar that can be life-threatening

8. _____ Evidence-based medicine

9. _____ Gastrointestinal

10. _____ Gross anatomy

11. _____ Hematology

12. _____ Microscopic anatomy

13. _____ Oncology

14. _____ Pathophysiology

A. prescribing medications for clinical use on the basis of scientific data

B. the study of structures within the body that are large enough to be seen by the naked eye

C. the study of structures within the body that can be seen with microscopes

D. the study of abnormal body functions that can be caused by disease or other abnormal processes

E. the study of cancerous diseases

F. the study of the blood

G. referring to digestive activities

15. _____ Pharmacology

16. _____ Physiology

17. _____ Pneumonia

18. _____ Receptors

19. _____ Respiratory

20. _____ Skeletal

A. referring to bones

B. the study of how drugs or other chemicals act in the body

C. the study of the functions within living things

D. minute specialized surfaces that provide the sites of actions for medications in different parts of the body

E. referring to lungs and other breathing passages

F. one type of infection that can be treated with anti-infective medications

Identify whether the following questions are true or false (circle one).

1. Accepted uses for medications are usually based on trial and error.
   TRUE   FALSE

2. Prescribing medications for clinical use on the basis of scientific data is termed *alternative medicine.*
   TRUE   FALSE

3. The science of medications is termed *anatomy*.
   TRUE   FALSE

4. Diabetes is a chronic condition associated with how the body processes sugar.
   TRUE   FALSE

5. Hematology medications are drugs that affect the muscles.
   TRUE   FALSE

6. Yoga is an example of a CAM.
   TRUE   FALSE

7. Receptors provide the sites of action for medications.
   TRUE   FALSE

8. The pharmacist is the health care professional who practices the science of pharmacy.
   TRUE   FALSE

9. Pharmacy technicians can assist pharmacists by performing routine tasks associated with preparing prescriptions for patients.
   TRUE   FALSE

10. The pharmacy technician performs drug utilization review, performs final checks on prescriptions, and counsels patients.
    TRUE   FALSE

STUDENT NAME _____

DATE _____ INSTRUCTOR'S NAME _____

Select the best available answer for the following questions.

1. Medications that are taken to treat sickness caused by infections. _____

    a. Respiratory medications
    b. Gastrointestinal medications
    c. Cardiovascular medications
    d. Anti-infective medications

2. High blood pressure is treated with _____.

    a. Respiratory medications
    b. Cardiovascular medications
    c. Reproductive medications
    d. Hematology medications

3. Oncology medications are used to treat _____.

    a. infections
    b. cancer
    c. diabetes
    d. nail fungus

4. Athlete's foot is treated with _____.

    a. oncology medications
    b. hematology medications
    c. muscular and skeletal medications
    d. dermatologic medications

5. Heartburn is treated with _____.

    a. cardiovascular medications
    b. hematology medications
    c. gastrointestinal medications
    d. respiratory medications

6. All of the following are examples of complementary and alternative medicine EXCEPT _____.

    a. prayer
    b. nutritional supplements
    c. pneumonia
    d. exercise

7. Which of the following is the scientific study of the structure of living things? _____

   a. anatomy
   b. physiology
   c. pathophysiology
   d. pharmacology

8. Pharmacists can perform all of the following activities EXCEPT _____.

   a. diagnosing diseases
   b. reviewing drug utilization
   c. medication counseling
   d. providing drug information

9. Pharmacy technicians can perform all of the following tasks EXCEPT _____.

   a. entering data into computers
   b. medication counseling
   c. managing inventory
   d. resolving insurance problems

10. In the typical medication dispensing process, the _____ performs drug utilization review.

    a. store clerk
    b. pharmacy technician
    c. pharmacist
    d. physician

Prescriptions, Medication Orders, and Legal Considerations

2

KEY TERMS

Behind-the-counter (BTC) drugs

Brand name

Controlled substances

Drug Enforcement Agency (DEA)

Food and Drug Administration (FDA)

Generic name

National Drug Code (NDC)

Over-the-counter (OTC) drugs

Poison Prevention Packaging Act (PPPA)

Third party

United States Adopted Names (USAN) Council

LEARNING OBJECTIVES

After completing this chapter, the student will be able to:

1. Explain the difference between prescriptions and medication orders
2. Describe what kinds of information are provided in a prescription
3. Describe what kinds of information are provided on a prescription label
4. Provide the meaning for abbreviations that are commonly used in prescriptions and medication orders
5. Differentiate between the FDA and DEA
6. List the five DEA schedules, which therapeutic categories are associated with the DEA schedules, and refill limitations associated with controlled substances
7. Describe the purpose of the Poison Prevention Packaging Act
8. List seven federal requirements for a prescription label
9. Identify the statement that is required on labels for controlled substances
10. Describe two differences between a generic name and a brand name
11. Describe the difference between OTC drugs and legend drugs

Introduction: How are Medications Regulated?

Medications are usually prescribed using prescriptions. When patients are in institutional settings, such as hospitals, medications are prescribed using medication orders. Pharmacists fill the prescriptions and medication orders in accordance with legal requirements. Knowing the following terms will be helpful as you learn about prescriptions and medication orders.

Behind-the-counter (BTC) drugs: drugs that can be purchased without a prescription but require documentation by the pharmacist

Controlled substances: drugs that are regulated by the DEA because of their potential for abuse

Drug Enforcement Agency (DEA): the federal agency that regulates controlled substances

Food and Drug Administration (FDA): the federal agency that approves drugs for sale in the United States

National Drug Code (NDC): a specific set of numbers assigned to a drug by the pharmaceutical company that produces it

Over-the-counter (OTC) drugs: drugs that can be purchased without a prescription

Poison Prevention Packaging Act (PPPA): a federal law that requires child-resistant closures on most prescription and nonprescription medications

Third party: prescription coverage through a patient's health care insurance

Prescriptions

To assist with filling a prescription, it is important for the pharmacy technician to have a basic understanding of what information is provided on the prescription blank.

In addition to the information provided on the sample prescription in Figure 2.1, additional information should also be obtained before the prescription is filled, including patient's date of birth, city and state of residence, zip code, and phone number. The original prescription date must be entered into the pharmacy computer record, and this is especially important for prescriptions for controlled substances.

The preprinted information on the prescription blank provides data about the prescriber of the medication and information about the patient and the medication that is to be received. In addition to handwritten prescriptions, prescriptions can be typed, computer generated, or transmitted electronically. Figure 2-1 shows a sample prescription that was written for patient Janet Smith by Dr. John Doe. The name of the medication prescribed is amoxicillin. The strength of the medication is 250 mg. The quantity to dispense is 30. The dosage is one capsule three times a day for 10 days. The pharmacy technician can assist the pharmacist in preparing the appropriate label for dispensing the prescription shown in Figure 2-2. Notice the prescription label provides all necessary information so that the patient can take the medication correctly. For this prescription, no refills were prescribed by the physician, and the label indicates that no refills are available.

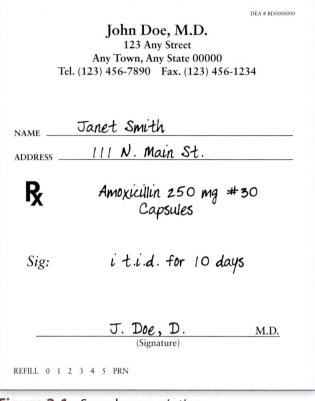

Figure 2-1. Sample prescription.

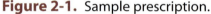

Figure 2-2. Sample label.

Medication Orders

In institutional settings, such as hospitals, medications are ordered, along with treatments and diagnostic procedures, in the patient's chart. The information needed to dispense medications for institutionalized patients is found in the section of the patient chart that contains physician's orders. The same kind of information is provided in a medication order as in a prescription: the name of the medication, the strength (for medications that are available in more than one strength), and the dosage. Patient information would include the patient's height and weight, as well as medication allergies.

Common Abbreviations Used in Prescriptions and Medication Orders

When interpreting prescriptions and medication orders, it is necessary to become familiar with standard terminology and abbreviations that are commonly used. Many of the abbreviations are based in Latin. Table 2-1 provides a list of some common abbreviations used in prescriptions along with their meanings.

Abbreviations should be used and interpreted carefully when preparing and filling prescriptions and medication orders. Medication errors are sometimes associated with abbreviations that are commonly used. The Institute for Safe Medication Practices

Table 2-1. Common Abbreviations Used in Prescriptions and Medication Orders

Abbreviation	Meaning	Abbreviation	Meaning	Abbreviation	Meaning
a.c.	before meals	o.d.	right eye	ss	one half
a.d.	right ear	o.s.	left eye	stat	immediately
a.s.	left ear	o.u.	both eyes	susp	suspension
a.u.	both ears	oint	ointment	sw	shake well
b.i.d.	twice daily	oz or ℨ	ounce	syr	syrup
C, cap	capsule	p.c.	after meals	T, tab	tablet
c.c.	with food *OR* cubic centimeter	p.m.	evening or afternoon	t.i.d.	three times a day
cr	cream	PO, p.o.	by mouth or orally	TPN	total parenteral nutrition
DAW	dispense as written (i.e., no generic substitution)	p.r.	by rectum	tbsp	tablespoon (15 ml)
		pfs	puffs	tr, tinc., tinct.	tincture
dc, D/C, disc	discontinue	PRN, p.r.n.	as needed	tsp or ℨ	teaspoon (5 ml)
g or gm	gram	q	every	u.d., u.t.d., u.t. dict.	as directed
gr	grain	q.4h	every 4 hours (replace "4" with other numbers accordingly)		
Gtt	drops			Ung	ointment
h, hr, or °	hour			Vag	vaginally
h.s.	at bedtime	q.a.m.	every day before noon	i	1
IM	intramuscular (with respect to injections)	q.d.	every day	ii	2
		q.h.	every hour	iii	3
IN	intranasal	q.h.s.	every night at bedtime	iv	4
IV	intravenous	q.i.d.	four times a day	v	5
IVP	intravenous push	q.o.d.	every other day	vi	6
IVPB	intravenous piggyback	q.p.m.	every day after noon	viii	8
liq	liquid	QS	quantity sufficient	x	10
mg	milligram	Sig	write on label	xii	12
non rep.	no repeats	SL	sublingually, under the tongue	xx	20
nr	no refills			xxx	30

Note: Abbreviations may appear in different forms from different health care professionals; some may use all capitals, some may use lowercase letters with periods to separate, and others may use a mixture of the two.

(ISMP) provides a listing of error-prone abbreviations (see Appendix G: http://www.ismp.org/tools/error proneabbreviations.pdf).

Prescriptions and Medication Orders for Controlled Substances

The dispensing of medications, whether in institutional settings or in community pharmacies, is regulated by federal and state law. Federal laws determine whether a medication can be obtained without a prescription. Drugs are approved in the United States by the Food and Drug Administration (FDA). Drugs that require a prescription are also known as legend drugs. Federal laws also determine whether a medication is a controlled substance.

Controlled substances are drugs that are regulated by the Drug Enforcement Agency (DEA) because of their potential for abuse. Controlled substances are classified by the DEA in five schedules: Schedules I, II, III, IV, and V. Prescribers must be currently registered with the DEA before they can order medications that are controlled substances. Similarly, pharmacies must be registered with the DEA before they can dispense medications that are controlled substances.

When filling prescriptions, one of the first considerations should be whether the medication is a controlled substance or not. Controlled substances have stricter requirements for record keeping, prescribing, refills, and labeling than noncontrolled substances.

Packaging and Labeling of Prescription Drugs

Most prescriptions for tablets and capsules are dispensed in amber vials with lids that provide a tight seal to protect the contents from environmental light or moisture. The Poison Prevention Packaging Act (PPPA) is a federal law intended to protect children from accidental poisoning. The PPPA requires child-resistant closures on most prescription and nonprescription drugs.

Federal laws require the following information on a prescription label:

℞ Name and address of pharmacy

℞ Name of patient

℞ Prescription number

℞ Name of prescriber

℞ Date (specific date requirements vary by state)

℞ Directions for use

℞ Any special cautionary statements for the patient (important for drugs that may cause drowsiness)

State laws may require other information on the prescription label. Some medications that have a limited shelf life should also contain a beyond use date for when the medication should no longer be used.

Additionally, labeling for prescriptions containing controlled substances must display the following statement: **CAUTION: Federal law prohibits the transfer of this drug to any other person than for whom it was prescribed.**

Third-party Billing

When prescriptions are filled in pharmacies, they are often billed to a third party. Third-party billing is associated with the patient's health care insurance. Most of the information required to fill the prescription, such as patient's name, date of birth, sex, prescription number, drug name and identifying code, quantity dispensed, and prescriber is also required for third-party billing. Additionally, a calculation for days supply is required for third-party billing.

Days Supply Calculations

A basic formula to calculate days supply is:

$$\text{Days supply} = \text{Amount of prescription} \div \text{amount per dose} \div \text{doses per day}$$

Examples:

Amoxicillin 250 mg #30, i cap t.i.d.
Amount of prescription = 30 capsules
Amount per dose = 1
Doses per day = 3

$$30 \div 1 \div 3 = 10 \text{ days supply}$$

Albuterol Syrup 120 ml, i ʒ q.i.d.
Amount of prescription = 120 ml
Amount per dose = i ʒ = 5 ml
Doses per day = 4

$$120 \text{ ml} \div 5 \div 4 = 6 \text{ days supply}$$

Brand and Generic Medications

When a prescriber orders a medication for a patient, the generic or brand name may be used. As noted in the previous chapter, a generic name is the single, specific name assigned to a drug by the United States Adopted Names (USAN) Council. In determining the generic names for drugs, USAN attempts to select simple, informative, and unique generic names for drugs using logical nomenclature classifications that are based on pharmacological and/or chemical properties of the drug. The ending "stems" of generic drug names represent the therapeutic category of the drug. The brand name is a unique name selected by a pharmaceutical company that produces the drug. The purpose of the brand name is to make it easy for prescribers to select and prescribe the drug product. The brand name is also known as the proprietary name. Every medication that has a brand name also has a generic name.

Brand and generic medications are identified by their National Drug Code (NDC) numbers. NDC numbers are assigned by the firms or pharmaceutical companies that produce the drugs and usually contain 10 digits separated into three segments. The first segment is the identifier for the firm that produces the drug. The second segment is the identifier for the drug and its strength. The third segment is the identifier for the package size or form. NDC numbers are commonly used for billing prescriptions to third parties. The FDA has a website for searching for NDC numbers by proprietary name, NDC number, active ingredient, firm name, or application number (http://www.access data.fda.gov/scripts/cder/ndc/default.cfm).

Nonprescription drugs

Over-the-counter (OTC) status is granted by the FDA for some medications that can be used safely without a prescription for conditions that can be self-diagnosed as long as the products have approved labeling. Federal law requires OTC medications to contain Drug Facts with the following recommended order:

1. Active ingredients
2. Purpose
3. Uses
4. Warnings
5. Directions
6. Other information (e.g., storage requirements)
7. Inactive ingredients

Another nonprescription category is behind-the-counter (BTC). BTC medications require documentation by the pharmacist, and the documentation must be kept on file. Examples of BTC medications include products containing pseudoephedrine.

Chapter Summary !

Medications are usually prescribed using prescriptions or medication orders. Pharmacy technicians can assist in the filling of prescriptions by interpreting the prescription and preparing the medication label. Technicians must be able to interpret common abbreviations and terminology. Federal and state laws dictate packaging and labeling requirements, as well as the level of control of a prescribed substance.

STUDENT NAME _____

DATE _____ INSTRUCTOR'S NAME _____

Match the following abbreviation with its meaning:

1. _____ b.i.d.
2. _____ o.u.
3. _____ q.a.m.
4. _____ h.s.
5. _____ IN
6. _____ nr
7. _____ p.o.
8. _____ qs

   A. Intranasal
   B. Bedtime
   C. No refills
   D. Quantity sufficient
   E. Twice daily
   F. Orally
   G. Both eyes
   H. Every day before noon

9. _____ DAW
10. _____ p.r.n.
11. _____ TPN
12. _____ ung
13. _____ p.m.
14. _____ p.c.
15. _____ p.r.
16. _____ q.i.d.

   A. Four times a day
   B. Dispense as written
   C. After meals
   D. Ointment
   E. Total parenteral nutrition
   F. By rectum
   G. As needed
   H. Evening or afternoon

17. _____ tbsp
18. _____ o.d.
19. _____ o.s.
20. _____ tsp
21. _____ vag
22. _____ oint
23. _____ oz
24. _____ sw

   A. Shake well
   B. Teaspoon
   C. Left eye
   D. Right eye
   E. Tablespoon
   F. Vaginally
   G. Ointment
   H. Ounce

25. _____ q		A.	Before meals
26. _____ a.d.		B.	Both ears
27. _____ mg		C.	Drops
28. _____ a.s.		D.	Left ear
29. _____ Sig		E.	Write on label
30. _____ a.c.		F.	Right ear
31. _____ gtt		G.	Every
32. _____ a.u.		H.	Milligram

33. _____ q.d.		A.	One half
34. _____ SL		B.	Sublingually, under the tongue
35. _____ q.4h.		C.	Every day
36. _____ q.p.m.		D.	Every other day
37. _____ q.h.s.		E.	Every hour
38. _____ q.h.		F.	Every day after noon
39. _____ q.o.d.		G.	Every four hours
40. _____ ss		H.	Every night at bedtime

41. _____ IV		A.	discontinue
42. _____ dc		B.	Intravenous piggyback
43. _____ C		C.	Intramuscular
44. _____ IVPB		D.	Capsule
45. _____ cr		E.	Intravenous
46. _____ IVP		F.	Cubic centimeter
47. _____ IM		G.	Intravenous push
48. _____ c.c.		H.	Cream

STUDENT NAME _____

DATE _____   INSTRUCTOR'S NAME _____

49. g	A. Grain
50. tr	B. Gram
51. u.t.d.	C. As directed
52. gr	D. No repeats
53. non rep.	E. Hour
54. liq	F. Drops
55. gtt	G. Liquid
56. h	H. Tincture

57. stat	A. Tincture
58. u.d.	B. Three times a day
59. tinc.	C. Suspension
60. t.i.d.	D. Immediately
61. susp	E. Tablet
62. syr	F. Puffs
63. T	G. As directed
64. pfs	H. Syrup

2. EXERCISES

Identify whether the following questions are true or false (circle one).

1. The PPPA requires that controlled substances be regulated.
    TRUE   FALSE

2. Medication orders are used in hospitals and may be contained in the patient's chart.
    TRUE   FALSE

3. Inactive ingredients must be listed on the prescription medication label.
    TRUE   FALSE

4. Prescription medication labels must contain the prescription number.
    TRUE   FALSE

5. Controlled substances are regulated by the FDA.
    TRUE   FALSE

6. Every medication that has a brand name also has a generic name.
    TRUE   FALSE

7. Medication dispensing is governed only by federal law.
    TRUE   FALSE

8. OTC medications require a prescription to be dispensed.
    TRUE   FALSE

9. Label requirements for an OTC medication include warnings and directions.
    TRUE   FALSE

10. Generic names for medications are assigned by the DEA.
    TRUE   FALSE

STUDENT NAME _____

DATE _____ INSTRUCTOR'S NAME _____

Select the best available answer for the following questions.

1. Pharmacies must be registered with the _____ before they can dispense medications that are controlled substances.

   a. FDA
   b. DEA
   c. PPPA
   d. USAN

2. Which of the following are not required on a prescription label according to federal law? _____

   a. Directions for use
   b. Name of prescriber
   c. Patient's date of birth
   d. Address of the pharmacy

3. A medication's brand name is selected by _____.

   a. the USAN
   b. the company that produces the drug
   c. the FDA
   d. the DEA

4. q.h.s. PRN means _____.

   a. every night at bedtime as needed
   b. every half hour as needed
   c. every day in the afternoon
   d. every hour in the afternoon

5. Which of the following means dispense as written? _____

   a. D.W.
   b. DAW
   c. u.t.d.
   d. D.T.W.

6. Controlled substances are classified in _____ schedules.

   a. Two
   b. Three
   c. Four
   d. Five

7. Legend drugs are also known as _____.

   a. prescription drugs
   b. OTC drugs
   c. controlled substances
   d. generic drugs

8. What does t.i.d. stand for? ____

    a. Total parenteral nutrition
    b. Tincture
    c. Three times daily
    d. Teaspoon

9. D/C is an abbreviation meaning ____.

    a. discontinue
    b. dispense in capsule form
    c. daily
    d. dispense in cream form

10. Calculate the days supply for the following prescription: Vicodin #24, i tab q.4h. ____

    a. 3
    b. 4
    c. 5
    d. 6

Basic Pharmacology and Dosage Forms

3

LEARNING OBJECTIVES

After completing this chapter, the student will be able to:

1. Describe how drugs interact at receptors
2. Differentiate between the terms *agonist, partial agonist*, and *antagonist*
3. Define the term *pharmacokinetics*
4. Explain ADME
5. Define routes of administration
6. Differentiate among IV, IM, and SQ routes of administration
7. Provide examples of drugs that are administered IV, IM, and SQ
8. Provide four examples of common side effects
9. Explain the time frame during which an anaphylactic reaction could occur
10. List the brand and generic names of 10 drugs with potentially serious drug interactions
11. Identify six dosage forms and state the appropriate route of administration for each

Introduction to Pharmacology

Most drugs work because of interactions that occur between the drug and receptors. Receptors are found throughout the body, and interactions with different receptors can produce different effects in different parts of the body.

Knowing the following terms will be helpful as you study some of the basic concepts of pharmacology.

Agonists: drugs that produce the desired effects when they interact with receptors

Anaphylactic shock: a severe, life-threatening hypersensitivity reaction; immediate emergency medical attention is necessary

Antagonists: drugs that block the effects of chemicals that would otherwise produce an effect through interaction with receptors

Carcinogenicity: drug effects that cause cancer

Drug interaction: effects that may result when a patient takes two drugs simultaneously

Hematological effects: drug effects that alter the composition of the blood

Hepatotoxicity: drug effects that damage the liver

Hypersensitivity: an allergic reaction

Intramuscular (IM): drug is injected into a muscle

Intravenous (IV): drug is injected directly into a vein

Nephrotoxicity: drug effects that damage the kidneys

Parenteral: route of administration other than the digestive system

Partial agonists: drugs that produce only partial effects through receptor interactions

Pharmacokinetics: the study of the absorption, distribution, metabolism, and excretion of drugs in the body after they are administered

Pharmacology: the study of how drugs or other chemicals work in the body

Receptors: minute specialized surfaces in different parts of the body that provide the sites of action for medications

Route of administration: the way a drug is administered

Side effects: unintended effects caused by a drug

Subcutaneous (SC, SQ): drug is injected into the fatty tissue just below the skin (note that the abbreviation for subcutaneous can be the source of medication errors)

Teratogenicity: drug effects that disrupt normal fetal development

One way to visualize how and why drugs produce their effects is to think of the interaction between drugs and receptors as similar to how a key opens a lock. Just as precisely designed keys that fit a given lock can open it, only certain drugs that fit a receptor can produce an effect through interaction at the receptor.

Many drugs interact at receptors in ways that compare with natural body chemicals.

Some drugs fit the receptor exactly, and when the drug interacts at the receptor, the full effect of the interaction is achieved. The drugs that produce the desired effects when they interact with the receptor are called agonists.

Other drugs have some interaction with the receptor but do not produce the full effect that is seen when an optimal fit is achieved. These drugs produce only partial effects through receptor interaction and are called partial agonists.

Some drugs stop chemicals found in the body from interacting with a receptor. These drugs block the effects of the chemicals and are called antagonists.

There are other ways that drugs can produce effects. One example is known as the placebo effect. A placebo is an agent that produces a response without having specific activity for the condition being treated. Other examples can be studied in more advanced pharmacology courses.

What is Pharmacokinetics?

Pharmacokinetics is a branch of pharmacology that studies what happens to medications in the body after they are administered. Pharmacokinetics includes the study of how drugs are absorbed and distributed in the body. It also includes the study of the rate of onset and duration of drug action, the metabolism of the drug including any chemical changes that occur to the drug in the body, and the excretion of the drug (i.e., how the body gets rid of the drug and its waste products). These processes are summarized by the abbreviation ADME, which stands for "absorption, distribution, metabolism, and excretion." The study of pharmacokinetics applies principles of chemistry and physics to help understand what happens to a drug after it has been administered. Using pharmacokinetic principles, drug dosing can be individualized. This is especially important for some drugs that have significant unwanted effects, called adverse effects or adverse reactions.

Routes of Administration

Drugs can be administered to patients in different ways. The most common and usually the easiest way is the oral route, in which tablets, capsules, or liquids are swallowed and enter the system through the digestive tract. Medications can also be dissolved in the mouth. Examples are sublingual medications that are dissolved under the tongue, buccal medications that are placed in the buccal pouch to be absorbed, film strips that dissolve on the tongue, and troches or lozenges that dissolve in the mouth. Some medications are not effective when taken orally and must be given parenterally. A parenteral medication is one that is administered through a route other than the digestive tract.

There are several routes of parenteral administration, but the four most common are intramuscular (IM), intravenous (IV), subcutaneous (SC), and topical. Medications administered through the intramuscular route are injected with a needle into a muscle. An example of a medication that is administered IM is the influenza vaccine. Medications administered intravenously are injected into a vein. An example of an IV medication is parenteral nutrition. Medications administered subcutaneously are injected into the fatty tissue under the skin. (Note the abbreviations for subcutaneous are sometimes the source of medication errors. For example, SC is sometimes mistaken as SL [sublingual] and SQ is sometimes mistaken as 5Q, or "5 every.") An example of a medication that is administered SC is insulin. Medications that are applied directly to the surface of the affected area are administered topically. Examples of topical medications are creams and ointments.

Intended Effects Versus Side Effects and Adverse Effects

Medications are administered for a specific intended effect. Along with the desired effects, medications have other effects that are not intended. The unintended effects are often called side effects or adverse effects. Side effects are generally uncomfortable or inconvenient, but not usually serious if they do not last long. Examples of common side effects are upset stomach, diarrhea, drowsiness, and dizziness. Most side effects do not require the patient to stop taking the medication. However, some side effects are considered serious and may require the patient to contact the prescriber and discontinue the medication. Pharmacy technicians should alert pharmacists when patients have questions about side effects.

Serious side effects can be related to unwanted effects on organs in the body, such as the liver or kidneys. The term for side effects affecting the liver is *hepatotoxicity*, and an example of a medication associated with hepatotoxicity is acetaminophen (Tylenol). The term for side effects affecting the kidney is *nephrotoxicity*, and an example of a medication associated with nephrotoxicity is ibuprofen (Motrin).

Drug dependence can also be considered a serious side effect. Chronic usage of some potent prescription pain relievers such as oxycodone (OxyContin) is associated with drug dependence.

Teratogenicity is another serious side effect. Teratogenicity is the ability of a drug to cause abnormal fetal development when taken by a pregnant woman.

Carcinogenicity is also a serious side effect. Carcinogenicity is the ability of a drug to cause cancer.

Some drugs cause effects on the composition of the blood. These are called hematological effects and can sometimes be serious.

Hypersensitivity is an example of a side effect that can be considered minor or serious, depending on the patient. Hypersensitivity is another name for allergic reaction. Some allergic reactions are not serious and cause only minor rashes accompanied by itching. However, other allergic reactions are serious and life-threatening. Anaphylactic shock is a serious side effect that can result in death. Anaphylactic shock occurs within minutes after exposure to the drug that causes the allergic reaction, and immediate treatment is necessary to prevent death.

Drug Interactions

Any time a patient takes more than one drug at a time, he or she can experience a drug interaction. A drug interaction occurs when the effects of one drug cause an increase or decrease in the effects of another drug. Drugs can also interact with herbal products, dietary supplements, and food or alcohol. Pharmacists develop an understanding of drug interactions when they are preparing to become a pharmacist. In practice, pharmacists are able to apply their knowledge and experience about drug interactions to make clinical decisions about drug therapy for patients who are taking multiple medications.

Pharmacy technicians should be aware of the importance of alerting the pharmacist when drug interactions are detected. A few examples of drugs with potentially serious drug interactions are shown in Table 3-1.

Dosage forms

The term *dosage form* describes the physical appearance of a medication, and the dosage form provides some indication of how a drug should be taken. Examples of common dosage forms are tablets, capsules, caplets, gel caps, oral suspensions, oral solutions, ophthalmic suspensions, ophthalmic solutions, otic suspensions, otic solutions, nasal sprays, inhalers, rectal suppositories, vaginal suppositories, parenteral solutions, parenteral suspensions, creams, ointments, and gels, as shown in Table 3-2.

Table 3-1. Examples of Some Drugs with Potentially Serious Drug Interactions

Generic Name	Brand Name (U.S.)	Generic Name	Brand Name (U.S.)
alprazolam	Xanax	lovastatin	Altoprev, Mevacor
amitriptyline	Elavil, Endep	methotrexate	Rheumatrex
atorvastatin	Lipitor	midazolam	No trade name in the United States
carbamazepine	Tegretol	olanzapine	Zyprexa
cimetidine	Tagamet	paroxetine	Paxil
ciprofloxacin	Ciloxan, Cipro	phenobarbital	Lumnal
clarithromycin	Biaxin	phenytoin	Dilantin
clozapine	Clozaril	quinidine	Cardioquin, Quinaglute
cyclosporine	Neoral, Sandimmune	rifabutin	Mycobutin
diazepam	Valium	rifampin	Rifadin, Rimactane
digoxin	Digitek, Lanoxin	ritonavir	Norvir
diltiazem	Cardizem, Cartia, Dilacor	sildenafil	Viagra
erythromycin	Ery-tab, Erythrocin	simvastatin	Zocor
fluconazole	Diflucan	tacrolimus	Prograf
fluoxetine	Prozac, Sarafem	tadalafil	Cialis
fluvoxamine	Luvox	telithromycin	Ketek
imipramine	Tofranil	theophylline	Elixophyllin, Theo-Dur
itraconazole	Sporanox	triazolam	Halcion
ketoconazole	Nizoral	vardenafil	Levitra
lithium	Eskalith, Lithobid, Lithonate	warfarin	Coumadin

Table 3-2. Common Dosage Forms and Their Common Routes of Administration

Mouth	Rectum
Tablets	Rectal suppositories
Capsules	Rectal solutions
Caplets	Rectal suspensions
Gel caps	**Urethra**
Film strips	Urethral suppositories
Lozenges or troches	**Vagina**
Oral inhalation capsules	Vaginal creams
Oral elixirs	Vaginal gels
Oral syrups	Vaginal ointments
Oral suspensions	Vaginal suppositories
Oral solutions	**Injection (read product information to determine if IM, IV, or SQ)**
Oral inhalers	
Eye	Parenteral solutions
Ophthalmic suspensions	Parenteral suspensions
Ophthalmic solutions	**Topical**
Ophthalmic ointments	Creams
Ear	Ointments
Otic suspensions	Gels
Otic solutions	Powders
Nose	
Nasal sprays	
Nasal inhalers	

Chapter Summary !

Some medications work similarly to a lock and key, with the medication (the key) working as an agonist, partial agonist, or antagonist at a receptor (the lock). Absorption, distribution, metabolism, and excretion are the foundation of pharmacokinetics, the branch of pharmacology that studies what happens to medications in the body after they are administered. Different dosage forms may be given in various ways, including oral, intravenous, and topical. Side effects, or unintended effects of a medication, may occur with medication use. Drug interactions may also occur if two or more medications are taken at once, even if by different routes of administration.

STUDENT NAME _____

DATE _____ INSTRUCTOR'S NAME _____

Match the following terms with their definitions:

1. _____ Carcogenicity
2. _____ Parenteral
3. _____ Agonists
4. _____ Hypersensitivity
5. _____ Receptors
6. _____ Side effects
7. _____ Pharmacokinetics
8. _____ Teratogenicity

A. Route of administration other than the digestive system
B. An allergic reaction
C. Minute specialized surfaces in different parts of the body that provide the sites of action for medications
D. Drug effects that cause cancer
E. A branch of pharmacology that studies what happens to medications in the body after they are administered
F. Drug effects that disrupt normal fetal development
G. Unintended effects caused by a drug
H. Drugs that produce the desired effects when they interact with receptors

9. _____ Intramuscular (IM)
10. _____ Intravenous (IV)
11. _____ Subcutaneous (SQ)
12. _____ Pharmacology
13. _____ Anaphylactic shock
14. _____ Route of administration
15. _____ Nephrotoxicity
16. _____ Hepatotoxicity

A. Drug effects that damage the kidneys
B. A severe, life-threatening hypersensitivity reaction; immediate emergency medical attention is necessary
C. Drug is injected into a muscle
D. Drug effects that damage the liver
E. Drug is injected directly into a vein
F. The way a drug is administered
G. The study of how drugs or other chemicals work in the body
H. Drug is injected into the fatty tissue just below the skin

17. _____ Antagonist
18. _____ Partial agonist
19. _____ Drug interaction
20. _____ Hematological effects

A. Drug effects that alter the composition of the blood
B. Effects that may result when a patient takes two drugs simultaneously
C. Drugs that block effects of other chemicals that would otherwise produce an effect through interaction with receptors
D. Drugs that produce only partial effects through receptor interactions

3. EXERCISES

Identify whether the following questions are true or false (circle one).

1. Parenteral suspensions can be given intravenously.
   TRUE OR FALSE

2. Tablets, caplets, and gel caps are all given by mouth.
   TRUE OR FALSE

3. Pharmacy technicians do not need to notify the pharmacist if a drug interaction is detected.
   TRUE OR FALSE

4. Anaphylactic shock is a minor condition, rarely requiring treatment.
   TRUE OR FALSE

5. Teratogenicity is an example of a serious side effect.
   TRUE OR FALSE

STUDENT NAME _____

DATE _____   INSTRUCTOR'S NAME _____

Select the best available answer for the following questions.

1. Agonists work by _____.
   a. producing only partial effects through receptor interaction
   b. blocking the effects of other chemicals
   c. producing the desired effects when they interact with receptors
   d. None of the above

2. ADME stands for _____.
   a. Administration, dispensing, marketing, and explaining concepts to patients
   b. Absorption, distribution, metabolism, and excretion
   c. Administration, distribution, microscopic anatomy, and excretion
   d. Absorption, dispensing, metabolism, and explaining concepts to patients

3. The most common and usually the easiest way medications are administered is through which route? _____
   a. Intravenous
   b. Intramuscular
   c. Oral
   d. Subcutaneous

4. Hepatotoxicity is a side effect that affects the _____, whereas nephrotoxicity is a side effect that affects the _____.
   a. Kidney; liver
   b. Liver; kidney
   c. Kidney; brain
   d. Brain; liver

5. Carcinogenicity is the ability of a drug to _____.
   a. cause a drug interaction
   b. cause cancer
   c. cause drug dependency
   d. cause abnormal fetal development

6. Hematological effects alter the _____.
   a. risk of drug interaction
   b. risk of cancer
   c. fetal development
   d. composition of the blood

7. Injections given by the _____ route are injected into the fatty tissue below the skin.
   a. IM
   b. IV
   c. SQ
   d. PO

8. Which of the following is not a common side effect? _____
    a. Upset stomach
    b. Diarrhea
    c. Drug dependence
    d. Drowsiness

9. If a patient has a question about a side effect, a pharmacy technician should _____.
    a. alert the pharmacist
    b. tell the patient that side effects are not a problem
    c. tell the patient to stop taking the medication
    d. tell the patient to go to the emergency room immediately

10. The appropriate route of administration of an otic solution is _____.
    a. ear
    b. eye
    c. nose
    d. mouth

Anti-infective and Other Immunologic Medications

4

KEY TERMS

Acquired immune deficiency syndrome (AIDS)

Antibacterial

Antibiotic

Antifungal

Antimicrobial

Antiviral

Bacteria

Benign tumor

Cancer

Fungus

Human immunodeficiency virus (HIV)

Immunization

Immunobiologic

Immunology

Malignant tumor

Pathogenic

Respiratory syncytial virus (RSV)

Tumor

Vaccination

Vaccine

Virus

LEARNING OBJECTIVES

After completing this chapter, the student will be able to:

1. Describe the basic anatomy and physiology of the immune system
2. Explain the therapeutic effects of common medications used to treat diseases of the immune system
3. List the brand and generic names of common medications used to treat diseases of the immune system
4. Identify available dosage forms for common immune system medications
5. Identify routes of administration for common immune system medications
6. Identify usual doses for common immune system medications
7. List common side effects of common immune system medications
8. Define medical terms commonly used when treating diseases of the immune system
9. List abbreviations for terms associated with use of medication therapy for common diseases affecting the immune system
10. Describe alternative therapies commonly used to treat diseases of the immune system

Basic Anatomy and Physiology of the Immune System

The immune system functions to spare people from diseases by identifying and killing pathogens and tumor cells. It is important for the immune system to be able to distinguish between disease-causing materials and the body's own healthy cells and tissues. Immunology includes the study of the immune system, especially in relation to health and disease.

Specifically, the lymphatic system is the term for the collection of tissues and organs that fight infection and disease. The bone marrow, spleen, thymus, tonsils, and lymph nodes (Figure 4-1), are important parts of the lymphatic

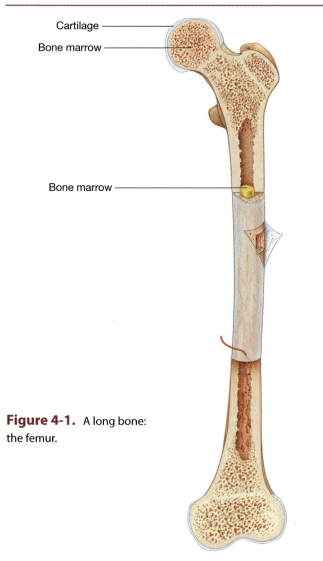

Cartilage
Bone marrow

Bone marrow

Figure 4-1. A long bone: the femur.

system. Figure 4-1 shows where the bone marrow could be found in a long bone, in this case the femur bone of the leg. Figure 4-2 shows the spleen, thymus, tonsils, and lymph nodes of the lymphatic system.

Disorders in the immune system can result in diseases ranging from bacterial, fungal, or viral infections to acquired immune deficiency syndrome (AIDS) and also cancerous tumors.

Knowing the following terms will be helpful as you learn about the medications used to treat conditions affecting the immune system.

Acquired immune deficiency syndrome (AIDS): A disease of the human immune system that makes the individual highly vulnerable to life-threatening diseases

Antibacterial: A substance able to inhibit or kill bacteria

Antibiotic: A substance able to inhibit or kill a microorganism

Antifungal: A substance able to inhibit or kill a fungus

Antimicrobial: A substance able to inhibit or kill a microorganism

Antiviral: A substance able to inhibit or kill a virus

Bacteria: Single-celled microorganisms that are often aggregated into colonies and may be pathogenic

Benign tumor: A mild type of abnormal new tissue growth that has no physiologic function and that does not threaten health

Cancer: A malignant tumor that has unlimited potential for growth

Fungus: A type of organism that was formerly classified as a plant without chlorophyll and includes molds, rusts, mushrooms, and yeasts

Human immunodeficiency virus (HIV): The virus that causes AIDS

Immunization: The creation of immunity to a particular disease through vaccination

Immunobiologic: An agent associated with the physiological reactions of the immune system

Immunology: The study of the immune system especially related to health and disease

Malignant tumor: A type of abnormal new tissue growth that has no physiologic function and that threatens health and can lead to death

Pathogenic: Capable of causing disease

Respiratory syncytial virus (RSV): A virus that causes serious lower respiratory tract infections in children and infants

Tumor: An abnormal new growth of tissue that possesses no physiological function

Vaccination: Administration of a microorganism that has been treated to make it harmless and will produce immunity to a disease

Vaccine: A preparation of microorganisms that have been treated to make them harmless that is administered to produce immunity to a disease

Virus: Any of a large group of submicroscopic agents that can cause infection

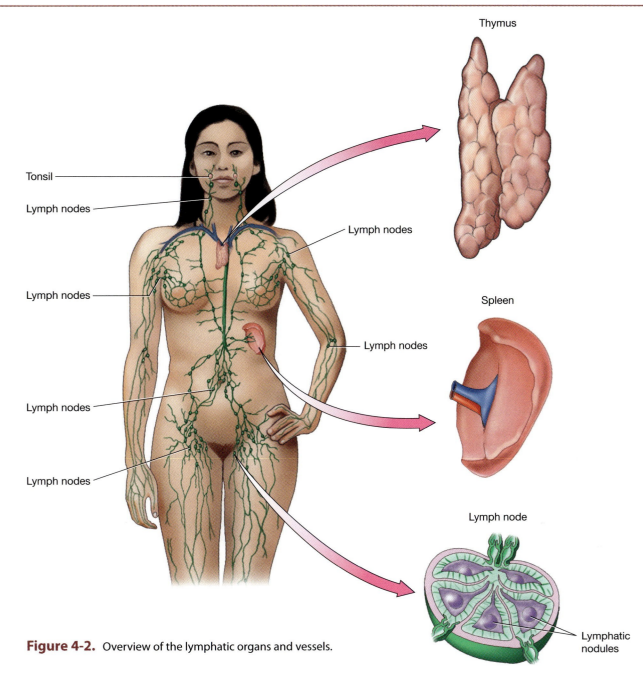

Figure 4-2. Overview of the lymphatic organs and vessels.

Primer on Pharmacologic Actions of Immunologic Agents

Immunologic medications are used to treat a wide variety of conditions associated with the immune system. These medications are used to treat bacterial, fungal, and viral infections, as well as AIDS and cancerous tumors. Additionally, immunobiologic agents such as vaccines can be used to prevent certain diseases.

Bacteria are single-celled microorganisms that are often aggregated into colonies and may be pathogenic. Diseases caused by pathogenic bacteria

sometimes require treatment with medications. Drugs used to treat bacterial infections are classified in the laboratory as bactericidal or bacteriostatic. Bactericidal agents kill bacteria directly, whereas bacteriostatic agents slow the growth of bacteria. Additionally, the drugs are classified according to their chemical structures. The most common antibiotic classifications are aminoglycosides, carbacephems, cephalosporins, glycopeptides, lincosamides, macrolides, nitrofurans, penicillins and penicillin combinations, polypeptides, quinolones, sulfonamides, and tetracyclines; there are also other commonly used agents that fall in other classes.

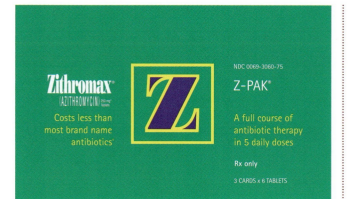

What is a common use for Zithromax?

A fungus is a type of organism that was formerly classified as a plant without chlorophyll and includes molds, rusts, mushrooms, and yeasts. Some types of fungus are pathogenic and can cause fungal infections. Common fungal infections include athlete's foot, ringworm, and candidiasis (thrush), as well as serious systemic infections. Drugs used to treat fungal infections are classified according to their chemical structures as polyene antifungals; imidazole, triazole, and thiazole antifungals; allylamines; and echinocandins. Additional agents also have antifungal activity. Antifungal drugs are usually obtained by a doctor's prescription, but some can be purchased over the counter.

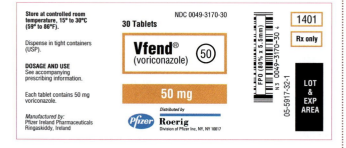

What is a common use for Vfend?

A virus is any of a large group of submicroscopic agents that can cause infection. Drugs used to treat viral infections include agents used for herpes infections (such as cold sores and genital herpes), hepatitis B, hepatitis C, influenza A, and influenza B. There are also other types of viral infections, including respiratory syncytial virus (RSV) and human immunodeficiency virus (HIV) viruses.

RSV is a virus that causes serious lower respiratory tract infections in children, especially in infants. Palivizumab (Synagis) is used to help prevent RSV.

HIV is a special type of virus that causes AIDS, a condition in which the immune system fails. Patients with AIDS can be susceptible to life-threatening bacterial, fungal, and viral infections. Drugs used to treat HIV and AIDS are a special category of antiviral agents. There is currently no cure for HIV or AIDS. The two largest classes of drugs used for HIV or AIDS are reverse transcriptase inhibitors and protease inhibitors. Drugs from other classes are also used to treat HIV and AIDS.

A tumor is an abnormal new growth of tissue that possesses no physiological function. Tumors can be characterized as benign or malignant. A benign tumor is a mild type of abnormal new tissue growth that has no physiologic function and that does not threaten health. A malignant tumor is more serious than a benign tumor; these tumors usually threaten health and can lead to death. Malignant tumors are also known as cancerous tumors. Information about drugs to treat cancer can be found in Chapter 14.

Immunobiologic drugs are agents associated with the physiological reactions of the immune system. Vaccines are the most commonly used immunobiologic drugs. Information about vaccines can be found in Chapter 15.

Some common anti-infective agents and their uses are listed in Table 4-1.

Table 4-1. Common Anti-infective Agents and Their Uses

Generic Name	Brand Name	Dosage Form	Route	Common Use	Common Frequency	Common Strengths
atazanavir	Reyataz	Capsule	PO	Anti-HIV	q.d.	100mg, 150mg, 200mg
darunavir	Prezista	Tablet	PO	Anti-HIV	b.i.d.	300mg
efavirenz, emtricitabine, tenofovir	Atripla	Tablet	PO	Anti-HIV	q.d.	600mg/200mg/300mg
emtricitabine, tenofovir	Truvada	Tablet	PO	Anti-HIV	q.d.	200mg/300mg
raltegravir	Isentress	Tablet	PO	Anti-HIV	b.i.d.	400mg
ritonavir	Norvir	Capsule, liquid	PO	Anti-HIV	b.i.d.	100mg, 80mg/ml
aztreonam	Azactam	Parenteral	IV	Antibiotic, carbapenem	q.6–12h	1g, 2g
ertapenem	Invanz	Parenteral	IV, IM	Antibiotic, carbapenem	q.d.	1g
imipenem, cilastatin	Primaxin	Parenteral	IV	Antibiotic, carbapenem	q.6h	250mg, 500mg, 1g
meropenem	Merrem	Parenteral	IV	Antibiotic, carbapenem	q.8H	1g
cefaclor	Ceclor	Capsule, tablet, liquid	PO	Antibiotic, cephalosporin	q.8–12h	250mg, 500mg, 125mg/5ml, 250mg/5ml
cefadroxil	Duricef	Capsule, tablet, liquid	PO	Antibiotic, cephalosporin	q.d., q.12h	500mg, 1g, 250mg/5ml
cephalexin	Keflex	Capsule, liquid	PO	Antibiotic, cephalosporin	q.6h	250mg, 500mg, 125mg/5ml, 250mg/5ml
cefazolin	Ancef	Parenteral	IV	Antibiotic, cephalosporin	q.6h	500mg, 1g
cefdinir	Omnicef	Capsule, liquid	PO	Antibiotic, cephalosporin	b.i.d.	300mg, 125mg/5ml, 250mg/5ml
cefepime	Maxipime	Parenteral	IV	Antibiotic, cephalosporin	q.8–12h	500mg, 1g, 2g
cefixime	Suprax	Tablet, liquid	PO	Antibiotic, cephalosporin	q.d., b.i.d.	400mg, 100mg/5ml
cefprozil	Cefzil	Tablet, liquid	PO	Antibiotic, cephalosporin	q.12h	250mg, 500mg, 125mg/5ml, 250mg/5ml
ceftazidime	Fortaz	Parenteral	IV	Antibiotic, cephalosporin	q.8–12h	500mg, 1g, 2g
ceftriaxone	Rocephin	Parenteral	IV, IM	Antibiotic, cephalosporin	q.2h	500mg, 1g, 2g

(Continued)

Table 4-1. Common Anti-infective Agents and Their Uses *(Continued)*

Generic Name	Brand Name	Dosage Form	Route	Common Use	Common Frequency	Common Strengths
cefuroxime	Ceftin	Tablet, liquid	PO	Antibiotic, cephalosporin	q.2h	250mg, 500mg, 125mg/5ml, 250mg/5ml
azithromycin	Zithromax	Tablet, liquid, parenteral	IV, PO	Antibiotic, macrolide	q.d.	250mg, 500mg, 100mg/5ml, 200mg/5ml
clarithromycin	Biaxin	Tablet, liquid	PO	Antibiotic, macrolide	q.2h	250mg, 500mg, 125mg/5ml, 250mg/5ml
erythromycin	Erythrocin	Tablet, capsule	PO	Antibiotic, macrolide	q6–12h	250mg, 500mg, 1g
clindamycin	Cleocin	Capsule, parenteral	PO, IV	Antibiotic, miscellaneous	Q.6–8h	150mg, 300mg, 450mg, 900mg
daptomycin	Cubicin	Parenteral	IV	Antibiotic, miscellaneous	q.d.	500mg
isoniazid	I.N.H.	Tablet	PO	Antibiotic, miscellaneous	q.d.	100mg, 300mg, 50mg/5ml
linezolid	Zyvox	Tablet, parenteral	PO, IV	Antibiotic, miscellaneous	q.2h	600mg
metronidazole	Flagyl	Tablet, capsule, parenteral	PO, IV	Antibiotic, miscellaneous	q.6–8h	375mg, 500mg, 750mg
mupirocin	Bactroban	Topical	Topical	Antibiotic, miscellaneous	t.i.d.	15g, 30g, 22g
vancomycin	Vancocin	Capsule, parenteral	PO, IV	Antibiotic, miscellaneous	q.12–24h	125mg, 250mg, 500mg, 1g, 1.5g, 2g
nitrofurantoin	Macrodantin, Macrobid	Capsule	PO	Antibiotic, nitrofuran	q.6–12h	50mg, 100mg
amoxicillin	Amoxil, Polymox	Tablet, capsule, liquid	PO	Antibiotic, penicillin	q.8–2h	250mg, 500mg, 125mg/5ml, 200mg/5ml, 250mg/5ml, 400mg/5ml
amoxicillin, clavulanate	Augmentin	Tablet, liquid	PO	Antibiotic, penicillin	q.8–12h	250mg, 500mg, 875mg, 125mg/5ml, 200mg/5ml, 250mg/5ml, 400mg/5ml, 600mg/5ml
ampicillin	Omnipen, Polycillin, Principen	Capsule, liquid, parenteral	PO, IV, IM	Antibiotic, penicillin	q.6h	250mg, 500mg, 1g, 2g, 125mg/5ml, 250mg/5ml,
ampicillin, sulbactam	Unasyn	Parenteral	IV, IM	Antibiotic, penicillin	q.6h	150mg, 300mg, 1.5g, 3g
dicloxacillin	Dynapen	Capsule	PO	Antibiotic, penicillin	q.6h	250mg, 500mg

(Continued)

Table 4-1. Common Anti-infective Agents and Their Uses *(Continued)*

Generic Name	Brand Name	Dosage Form	Route	Common Use	Common Frequency	Common Strengths
penicillin G	Bicillin L-	Parenteral	IV, IM	Antibiotic, penicillin	Single dose	1.2 million units, 2.4 million units
penicillin V potassium	V-Cillin K, Veetids	Tablet, liquid	PO	Antibiotic, penicillin	b.i.d.-QID	250mg, 500mg, 250mg/5ml
piperacillin, tazobactam	Zosyn	Parenteral	IV, IM	Antibiotic, penicillin	q.6–8h	2.25g, 3.375g, 4.5g
ticarcillin, clavulanate	Timentin	Parenteral	IV	Antibiotic, penicillin	q.4–8h	3.1g
ciprofloxacin	Cipro	Tablet, parenteral	PO, IV	Antibiotic, quinolone	q.8–12h	200mg, 250mg, 400mg, 500mg, 750mg
levofloxacin	Levaquin	Tablet, parenteral	PO, IV	Antibiotic, quinolone	q.d.	500mg, 750mg
moxifloxacin	Avelox	Tablet, parenteral	PO, IV	Antibiotic, quinolone	q.d.	400mg
trimethoprim, sulfamethoxazole	Bactrim, Septra	Tablet, liquid, parenteral	PO, IV	Antibiotic, sulfonamide	q.6–12h	800/160mg, 400/80mg, 200/40mg/5ml
doxycycline	Vibramycin	Tablet, capsule, liquid, parenteral	PO, IV	Antibiotic, tetracycline	b.i.d.	50mg, 75mg, 100mg, 25mg/5ml
minocycline	Minocin	Capsule, tablet, parenteral	PO, IV	Antibiotic, tetracycline	b.i.d.	50mg, 75mg, 100mg
tetracycline	Sumycin	Capsule, tablet, liquid	PO	Antibiotic, tetracycline	q.6h	250mg, 500mg, 125mg/5ml
amikacin	Amikin	Parenteral	IV, IM	Antibiotics, aminoglycoside	q.8–24h	250mg
gentamicin	Gentak	Parenteral	IV, IM	Antibiotics, aminoglycoside	q.8–24h	100mg
streptomycin	Streptomycin	Parenteral	IM	Antibiotics, aminoglycoside	q.2h	1g
tobramycin	Tobrex	Parenteral	IV, IM	Antibiotics, aminoglycoside	q.8–24h	100mg
amphotericin B	AmBisome, Amphocin	Parenteral	IV	Antifungal	q.d.	50mg
butenafine	Mentax	Topical	Topical	Antifungal	q.d.–b.i.d.	1% cream
caspofungin	Cancidas	Parenteral	IV	Antifungal	q.d.	50mg, 70mg
ciclopirox	Loprox, Penlac	Topical	Topical	Antifungal	b.i.d.	0.77% gel, 0.77% cream, 1% shampoo, 8% solution

(Continued)

Table 4-1. Common Anti-infective Agents and Their Uses *(Continued)*

Generic Name	Brand Name	Dosage Form	Route	Common Use	Common Frequency	Common Strengths
fluconazole	Diflucan	Tablet, liquid, parenteral	PO, IV	Antifungal	q.d.	50mg, 100mg, 150mg, 200mg, 10mg/ml, 40mg/ml
itraconazole	Sporanox	Capsule, liquid	PO	Antifungal	q.d.–t.i.d.	100mg, 10mg/ml
ketoconazole	Nizoral	Tablet, topical	PO, topical	Antifungal	q.d.	200mg, 400mg, 2% cream, 1% shampoo
miconazole	Monistat 1, Monistat 3, Monistat 7	Topical	Intravaginally	Antifungal	q.d.	100mg, 200mg, 1200mg
nystatin	Mycostatin	Liquid, topical	PO, topical	Antifungal	b.i.d.–t.i.d.	100,000U-1,000,000U
terbinafine	Lamisil	Topical	Topical	Antifungal	b.i.d.	250mg, 500mg
terconazole	Terazol	Topical	Topical	Antifungal	q.d.	0.4% cream, 0.8% cream
acyclovir	Zovirax	Capsule, tablet, liquid, parenteral, topical	PO, IV	Antiviral	q.4–8h	200mg, 400mg, 500mg, 800mg, 1000mg, 200mg/5ml, 5%
amantadine	Symmetrel	Tablet, capsule, liquid	PO	Antiviral	b.i.d.	100mg, 50mg/5ml
oseltamivir	Tamiflu	Capsule, liquid	PO	Antiviral	q.d.–b.i.d.	30mg, 45mg, 75mg, 12mg/ml
palivizumab	Synagis	Parenteral	IM	Antiviral	q.month	100mg/ml
valacyclovir	Valtrex	Capsule	PO	Antiviral	q.d.–t.i.d.	500mg, 1000mg
zanamivir	Relenza	Inhaled	Inhaled	Antiviral	q.d.–b.i.d.	5mg
immune globulin	Carimune, Gamunex	Parenteral	IV	Treatment of immunodeficiency syndromes	q.3–4weeks	3g, 6g, 12g

Dosage Forms, Routes of Administration, and Usual Doses for Common Anti-infective Medications

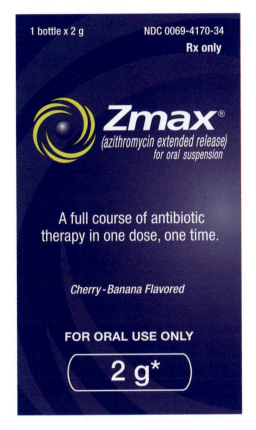

What is the proper route of administration for Zmax?

Capsules and tablets are common dosage forms for antibiotics, particularly when a patient is not in the hospital and is able to swallow pills. Younger children often require liquid formulations of antibiotics, specifically suspensions. Some antibiotics, such as penicillin G, are given intramuscularly. This allows a health care provider to give the injection in an outpatient office, and in some cases, the infection may be relieved with a single dose.

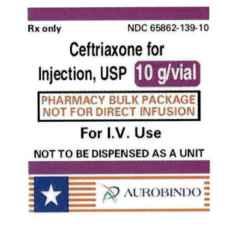

What is a common use for Ceftriaxone?

Intravenous anti-infectives are common in the hospital setting. In some instances, standard doses are given as part of a protocol for a condition, such as open heart surgery, to prevent infection. This can be considered preventive or prophylactic use. Other times, doses are calculated based on a patient's weight, age, or kidney function. Intravenous anti-infectives are occasionally given by a home health nurse if a patient is healing at home.

Technician Tip

Some anti-infectives are available in the community pharmacy as powders for re-constitution. These medications require that water be added by the pharmacy staff before dispensing. ℞

Common Side Effects of Anti-infective Medications

One of the most common side effects of anti-infectives is an upset stomach. Although an upset stomach is often remedied by eating a small snack or meal with the dose, this can be inappropriate with some anti-infectives that need to be taken on an empty stomach. Erythromycin is used therapeutically to increase the movement in a patient's gastrointestinal (GI) tract; therefore, it is an example of an antibiotic for which an upset stomach would be of special concern.

Some anti-infectives cause lower GI tract issues, such as diarrhea. Particularly in infants and small children, amoxicillin/clavulanate is widely known to cause diarrhea. Some health care providers will instruct the caregiver to change the types of foods fed to the child in an effort to combat the potential for diarrhea.

On occasion, after an anti-infective clears one infection, a second infection can begin almost immediately. For example, sometimes when a urinary tract infection is treated with an anti-infective, a yeast infection can follow. When this is of concern, it is important for the patient to be aware of this potential so that he or she can watch for signs and symptoms of a second infection.

Technician Tip

Some patients will say that they have an allergy to a medication when they may have an intolerance to it. An upset stomach following the use of an antibiotic is an example of an intolerance or side effect, but not an allergy. If there is any confusion as to whether a person is truly allergic to a medication or has an allergy, consult your pharmacist. ℞

Terminology and Common Abbreviations Used with Anti-infective Medications

See Table 2-1, page 13, for abbreviations.

What's in a name?

Table 4-2. Examples of USAN Stems for Anti-infective Medications		
Stem	**Description**	**Example**
-bactam	Beta-lactamase inhibitors	sulbactam
Cef-	Cephalosporins	cefaclor
-cillin	Penicillins	amoxicillin
-cycline	Antibiotics (tetracycline derivatives)	doxycycline
-oxacin	Antibacterials (quinolone derivatives)	ciprofloxacin

Sample Prescription for Anti-infective Medications

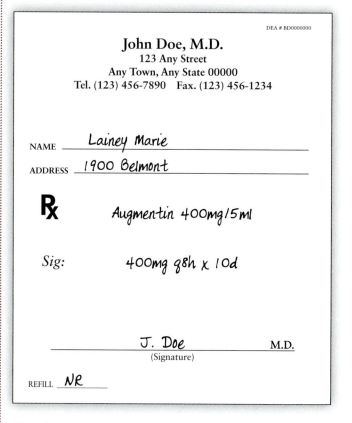

DEA # BD0000000

John Doe, M.D.
123 Any Street
Any Town, Any State 00000
Tel. (123) 456-7890   Fax. (123) 456-1234

NAME ___Lainey Marie___

ADDRESS ___1900 Belmont___

℞   Augmentin 400mg/5ml

Sig: 400mg q8h x 10d

_____ J. Doe _____ M.D.
(Signature)

REFILL ___NR___

The above prescription should be interpreted as Augmentin (amoxicillin and clavulanate) 400mg/5ml suspension, one teaspoonful (5ml) every eight hours for 10 days; 150ml should be dispensed.

Technician Tip

Amoxicillin/clavulanate (Augmentin) comes in several strengths, often listed and discussed by the amount of amoxicillin in the product. However, the amount of clavulanate does not always correspond between dosage forms. Be careful when calculating conversions to dispense different strengths when using amoxicillin/clavulanate. ℞

Technician Tip

Several antibiotics are dispensed as suspensions. Suspensions contain drug particles in the liquid that tend to settle; therefore, it is important to shake the stock bottle well before pouring the medication into the bottle for dispensing. It is also important for the patient to shake the bottle well before giving the dose. ℞

Additional Therapies for Infections

It is important to understand that anti-infectives rarely provide immediate relief of symptoms. It can take several days for a patient to feel improvement from antibiotics. Meanwhile, other medications may be required to reduce fever, decrease pain, clear a stuffy nose, or mediate other symptoms associated with the infection. Supportive care can also include maintaining good fluid intake, eating foods that do not upset the stomach, and reducing physical activity.

Chapter Summary !

Anti-infective medications can be used to treat a variety of bacterial, viral, and fungal infections in the outpatient and inpatient settings. Several categories of agents are available to treat various infectious sources.

℞ Antibiotics are commonly used to treat bacterial infections. Although many antibiotics are available in oral formulations, several others are available for intravenous administration for use in the hospital setting

℞ Antivirals are used to treat viral infections, such as RSV and herpes

℞ Antifungals can be given to treat fungal infections. Sometimes these are oral medications, but other antifungals are given topically. Fungal infections include thrush and athlete's foot

℞ Dispense the medications

Side effects, such as upset stomach and diarrhea, may have an impact on a patient's ability or willingness to take anti-infective medications. However, anti-infectives represent a common category of medications used in both inpatient and outpatient pharmacies.

3. How many refills are given on this prescription?

_____

_____

_____

_____

4. What other common strengths are available for Cipro?

_____

_____

_____

_____

5. How is this medication commonly categorized?

_____

_____

_____

_____

6. What is the days supply for this prescription?

_____

_____

_____

_____

STUDENT NAME _____

DATE _____ INSTRUCTOR'S NAME _____

DEA # BD0000000

John Doe, M.D.
123 Any Street
Any Town, Any State 00000
Tel. (123) 456-7890   Fax. (123) 456-1234

NAME   _Sarah Mathison_____

ADDRESS   _5514 McCoy Rd._____

Rx   Diflucan 150mg # 1

Sig: T 1 T PO now

_____   J. Doe   M.D.
(Signature)

REFILLS   NR _____

---

12 Cards x 1 Tablet   NDC 0049-3500-79

Rx only

Diflucan 150-mg
(fluconazole tablet)

Pfizer Roerig
Division of Pfizer Inc, NY, NY 10017

---

1. What is the generic name for Diflucan?

   _____

   _____

2. How would you translate the Sig code to plain English so that the patient could understand the directions for use?

   _____

   _____

   _____

3. How many refills are given on this prescription?

    _____

    _____

    _____

    _____

4. What other common strengths are available for Diflucan oral tablets?

    _____

    _____

    _____

    _____

5. How is this medication commonly categorized?

    _____

    _____

    _____

    _____

Cardiovascular Medications

5

KEY TERMS

Alpha-blocker

Angina

Angiotensin

Angiotensin converting enzyme (ACE)

Angiotensin II

Angiotensin II receptor blocker (ARB)

Anticoagulant

Antihypertensive

Arrhythmia

Arteries

Atherosclerosis

Bad cholesterol

Beta-blocker

Bile

Bile acid resin

Blood vessels

Calcium channel blocker (CCB)

Cardiovascular system

Good cholesterol

Congestive heart failure

Diuretic

Hyperlipidemia

Hypertension

Lipid

Lipoprotein

Protein

Thrombolytic

Vasodilator

Veins

LEARNING OBJECTIVES

After completing this chapter, the student will be able to:

1. Describe the basic anatomy and physiology of the cardiovascular system

2. Explain the therapeutic effects of common medications used to treat diseases of the cardiovascular system

3. List the brand and generic names of common medications used to treat diseases of the cardiovascular system

4. Identify available dosage forms for common cardiovascular system medications

5. Identify routes of administration for common cardiovascular system medications

6. Identify usual doses for common cardiovascular system medications

7. List common side effects of frequently prescribed cardiovascular system medications

8. Define medical terms commonly used to treat diseases of the cardiovascular system

9. List abbreviations for terms associated with use of medication therapy for common diseases affecting the cardiovascular system

10. Describe alternative therapies commonly used to treat diseases of the cardiovascular system

Basic Anatomy and Physiology of the Cardiovascular System

The cardiovascular system includes the heart and the blood vessels. It serves to transport oxygen and nutrients as well as other necessary substances and waste materials throughout the body. The heart is a sophisticated organ that provides the pumping force so that blood can travel through the blood vessels.

Figure 5-1 shows the anterior view, posterior view, and frontal section of the heart.

There are two main types of blood vessels: arteries and veins. Arteries can be thought of as a closed system of tubes that take oxygenated, nutrient-rich blood away from the heart and to organs and tissues.

Figure 5-2 shows the following major arteries of the body: right internal carotid artery, vertebral artery, right subclavian artery, brachiocephalic trunk (artery), aortic arch, ascending aorta, axillary artery, celiac trunk, brachial artery, abdominal aorta, suprarenal artery, radial artery, ulnar artery, palmar arches,

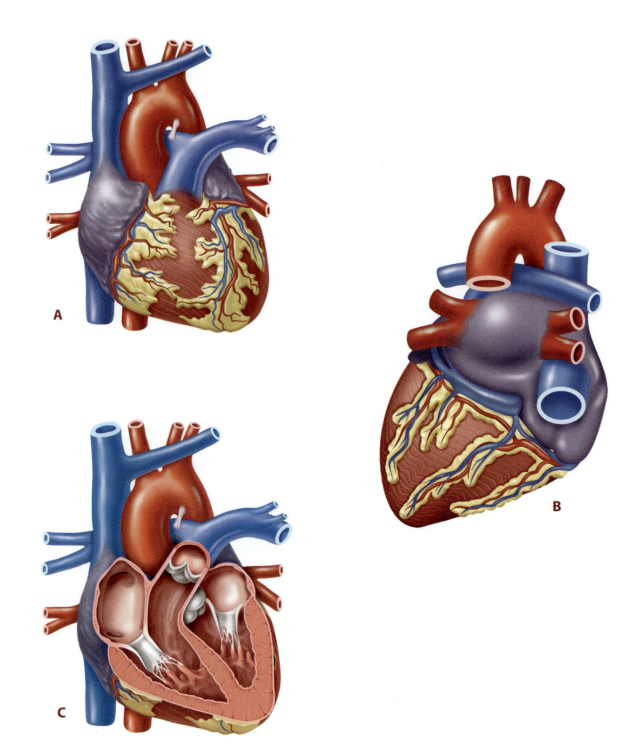

Figure 5-1. The heart: (**A**) anterior view; (**B**) posterior view; (**C**) frontal section.

external iliac artery, popliteal artery, posterior tibial artery, anterior tibial artery, plantar arch, temporal artery, right external carotid artery, right common carotid artery, left common carotid artery, left subclavian artery, axillary artery, pulmonary trunk, descending aorta, diaphragm, renal artery, superior mesenteric artery, gonadal artery, inferior mesenteric artery, common iliac artery, internal iliac artery, deep femoral artery, femoral artery, and dorsalis pedia artery. In contrast, veins transport deoxygenated, carbon dioxide-rich blood back toward the heart.

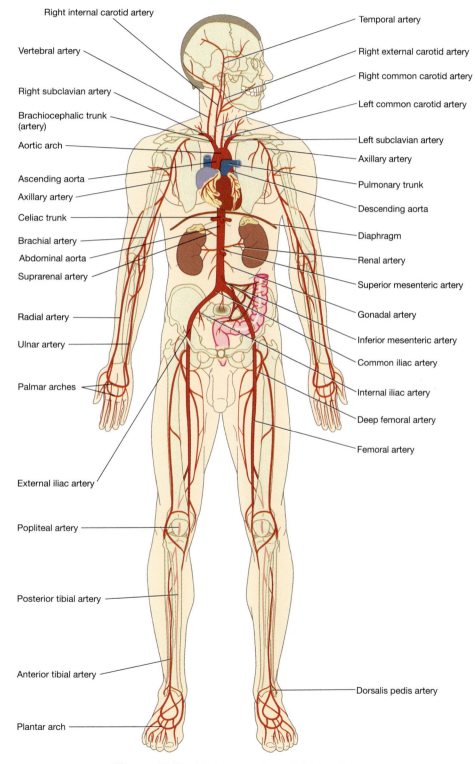

Figure 5-2. Major arteries of the body.

Figure 5-3 shows the location of the following major veins of the body: dural sinuses, vertebral vein, external jugular vein, subclavian vein, axillary vein, cephalic vein, brachial vein, basilica vein, hepatic veins, median cubital vein, radial vein, median antebrachial vein, ulnar vein, palmar venous arches, great saphenous vein, popliteal vein, small saphenous vein, plantar venous arch, dorsal venous arch, internal jugular vein, brachiocephalic vein, superior vena cava, intercostals veins, inferior vena cava, renal vein, gonadal vein, left and right common iliac veins, external iliac vein, internal iliac vein, deep femoral vein, femoral vein,

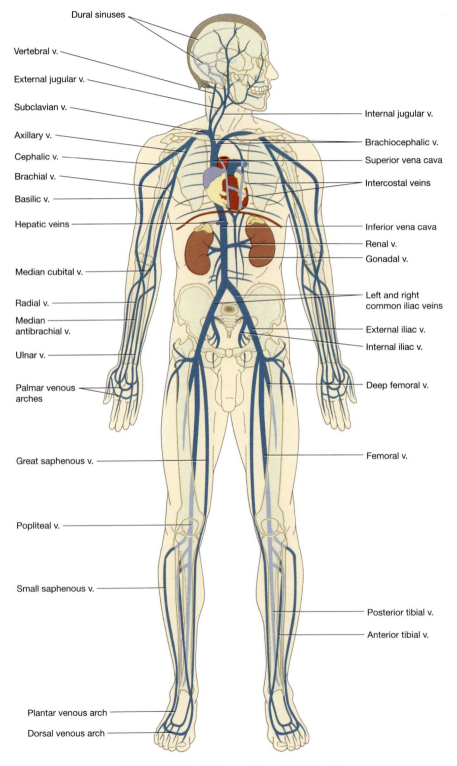

Figure 5-3. Major veins of the body.

posterior tibial vein, and anterior tibial vein. Blood vessels allow blood to circulate throughout the body.

Because the cardiovascular system is found throughout the body, disorders of this system can have broad effects. Such disorders can result in diseases including high blood pressure (hypertension), hyperlipidemia, atherosclerosis, along with a number of heart diseases, such as arrhythmias and congestive heart failure, angina, and other heart conditions.

Knowing the following terms will be helpful as you learn about the medications used to treat conditions affecting the cardiovascular system.

Alpha-blocker: a drug that combines with alpha-receptors and blocks the activity of alpha receptors

Angina: a disease marked by attacks of intense chest pain

Angiotensin: a protein that causes vasoconstriction

Angiotensin converting enzyme (ACE): an enzyme that converts angiotensin I to the active form angiotensin II

Angiotensin II: the active form of angiotensin

Angiotensin II receptor blocker (ARB): a drug that blocks the vasoconstriction caused by angiotensin II

Anticoagulant: a drug that hinders coagulation of the blood

Antihypertensive: a drug that is used to treat high blood pressure

Arrhythmia: a condition in which the heartbeat is altered

Arteries: blood vessels that carry blood rich in nutrients and oxygen away from the heart and throughout the body

Atherosclerosis: condition caused by a buildup of fatty materials such as cholesterol in the walls of arteries, causing the artery walls to thicken

Bad cholesterol: a lipoprotein in the blood that is associated with increased likelihood of developing atherosclerosis (low-density lipoprotein, LDL)

Beta-blocker: a drug that combines with beta-receptors to block the activity of a beta-receptor, decreasing the heart rate and forcing contractions of the heart

Bile: a fluid produced by the liver and passed into the digestive system that aids with digestion and the processing of cholesterol and other fats

Bile acid resin: medications that bind with certain components of bile in the gastrointestinal tract and can aid in lowering cholesterol

Blood vessels: closed system of tubes in the body that circulate blood

Calcium channel blocker (CCB): drug that blocks calcium channels in the muscle cells of the heart and blood vessels to prevent calcium from entering these cells, resulting in reduced blood pressure

Cardiovascular system: the organ system that distributes blood throughout the body

Good cholesterol: a lipoprotein in the blood that is associated with decreased likelihood of developing atherosclerosis (high-density lipoprotein, HDL)

Congestive heart failure: a condition in which the heart is unable to maintain adequate circulation of blood in the body

Diuretic: a drug that increases urination and lowers blood pressure

Hyperlipidemia: a condition of excess lipids in the blood

Hypertension: abnormally high blood pressure

Lipid: non-water-soluble substances such as fats that are important in the body

Lipoprotein: proteins that conjugate with lipids

Protein: naturally occurring complex substances that include many essential biological compounds such as enzymes, hormones, and antibodies

Thrombolytic: a drug that breaks down blood clots

Vasodilator: a drug that causes blood vessels to dilate

Veins: blood vessels that carry blood toward the heart

Primer on Pharmacologic Actions of Cardiovascular Agents

Cardiovascular medications can generally be thought of as drugs that affect the heart and blood vessels. The most common cardiovascular conditions are hypertension, angina, hyperlipidemia, and heart disease. Treatment of hypertension and hyperlipidemia can prevent further complications of some heart diseases. Anticoagulant medications are drugs that prevent blood clots from forming, and thrombolytic medications are drugs used to treat conditions associated with blood clots that have already formed.

Antihypertensive Agents

Hypertension is a common disorder, and there are many drugs available for its treatment.

The most common classes of antihypertensive agents are diuretics, beta-blockers, angiotensin converting enzyme (ACE) inhibitors, angiotensin antagonists, calcium channel blockers (CCBs), alpha-blockers, alpha/beta-blockers, nervous system inhibitors, and vasodilators. Antihypertensive drugs are most commonly used to treat hypertension; however, many of these agents have a wide range of uses, which vary according to the agent but commonly include angina, migraine headaches, and heart arrhythmias.

Diuretics reduce blood pressure through action in the kidney and remove excess water and sodium from the body. Diuretics are sometimes called "water pills." Furosemide (Lasix) is an example of a diuretic.

Beta-blockers affect nerve conduction in the heart and blood vessels and cause the heart to beat more slowly and with less force. Beta-blockers cause a decrease in blood pressure and also decrease the work of the heart. They are useful to treat hypertension, angina, and heart arrhythmias. Propranolol (Inderal) and metoprolol (Lopressor) are examples of beta-blockers.

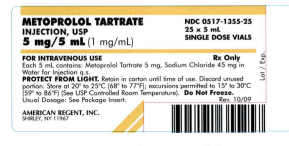

What is a common use for metoprolol?

ACE inhibitors prevent the formation of angiotensin. Angiotensin is a hormone that causes blood vessels to narrow. Therefore, ACE inhibitors cause blood vessels to relax and blood pressure to decrease. Enalapril

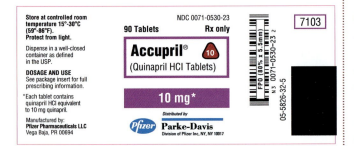

(Vasotec) and Accupril (quinapril) are examples of ACE inhibitors.

Angiotensin antagonists block the effects of angiotensin II on blood vessels. Angiotensin antagonists are also known as angiotensin blockers (ARB). Angiotensin II is a hormone that causes blood vessels to narrow. Therefore, ARBs also cause blood vessels to relax and blood pressure to decrease. An example of an ARB is valsartan (Diovan).

CCBs block calcium channels in the muscle cells of the heart and blood vessels to prevent calcium from entering these cells. The result of blocking the calcium channels is to relax blood vessels and reduce blood pressure. CCBs are used for other conditions, including angina and some cardiac arrhythmias. Verapamil (Calan, Isoptin) is an example of a calcium channel blocker.

Alpha-blockers are drugs that reduce nerve conduction to blood vessels. The actions of alpha-blockers cause a reduction in blood pressure. Some alpha-blockers are also used to treat benign prostatic hyperplasia (BPH). An example of an alpha-blocker is terazosin (Hytrin). More information about the use of alpha-blockers for BPH can be found in Chapter 11.

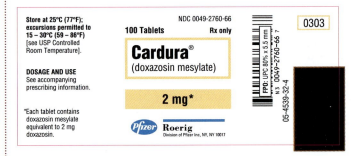

How is Cardura administered?

Alpha/beta-blockers reduce blood pressure in the same way as alpha-blockers, but they also slow the heart rate. An example of an alpha/beta-blocker is carvedilol (Coreg).

Nervous system inhibitors also act to control nerve conduction. The actions of nervous system inhibitors cause blood pressure to decrease.

Vasodilators are drugs that relax the muscles in the walls of blood vessels. The actions of vasodilators cause a decrease in blood pressure.

Antianginal Agents

Angina is a disease of the heart characterized by spasmodic attacks of intense chest pain. The most common drug used to treat angina is nitroglycerin. There are different dosage forms of nitroglycerin. Some dosage forms are used to prevent angina attacks from occurring. Other forms are used to treat acute attacks of angina. Nitroglycerin (Nitrostat) is an example of a drug used for acute angina attacks.

Antihyperlipidemic Agents

Antihyperlipidemic agents are medications used to reduce the amount of bad cholesterol in the blood. High levels of bad cholesterol increase the chances of developing heart disease. Bad cholesterol buildup in the arteries can lead to atherosclerosis or hardening of the arteries. Too much bad cholesterol can also increase the risk of heart attacks. The most common classes of antihyperlipidemic agents are statins, bile acid resins, ezetimibe, nicotinic acid, and fibrates.

The most common type of drug used to lower blood bad cholesterol are the statins, so-called because their generic names end in -statin. Statins work in the liver and block an enzyme that controls the synthesis of cholesterol. Statins have other effects in the liver that affect the levels of different kinds of cholesterol that circulate in the blood. One example of a statin is lovastatin (Mevacor).

Bile acid resins are drugs that bind with bile acids in the intestine so that the acids are eliminated in the feces. Bile acids are important because they contain cholesterol, so their removal provides a way to remove bad cholesterol from the system as well. Cholestyramine (Questran) is an example of a bile acid resin.

Ezetimibe (Zetia) is a drug that decreases the amount of bad cholesterol that is absorbed in the diet.

Nicotinic acid (niacin) is a type of vitamin B that can be prescribed by a physician in high doses to cause a reduction in bad cholesterol.

Fibrates are drugs that reduce only some forms of bad cholesterol. One commonly prescribed fibrate is gemfibrozil (Lopid).

Anticoagulant agents are drugs that prevent blood clots from forming. They are sometimes called "blood thinners." The two most common anticoagulants are warfarin (Coumadin) and heparin.

Warfarin is an oral medication used to prevent blood clots from forming and is prescribed for patients with certain arrhythmias and artificial heart valves. It is often prescribed for patients who have recently had a heart attack.

Heparin is an injectable medication used to prevent blood clots from forming and is prescribed for patients with some medical conditions, as well as for patients undergoing certain medical procedures that are associated with an increase of clot formation. Heparin is also used to stop the growth of clots that have already formed in the blood vessels and, in small amounts, to prevent blood clots from forming in catheters. For some patients, heparin cannot be used because it causes complications, and substitute anticoagulants such as hirudin or argatroban may be given.

Thrombolytic Agents

Thrombolytic agents are clot-busting drugs used immediately following a heart attack or stroke. The most common thrombolytic agent is tissue plasminogen activator (tPA).

In addition to the broad categories just described, numerous other cardiovascular agents are prescribed to treat a wide variety of cardiovascular conditions. See Tables 5-1 and 5-2.

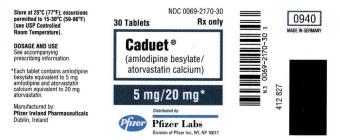

What are the two main uses for Caduet?

Some common cardiovascular agents and their uses are listed in Table 5-1.

Table 5-1. Common Cardiovascular Agents and Their Uses

Generic Name	Brand Name	Dosage Form	Route	Common Use	Common Frequency	Common Strengths
benazepril	Lotensin	Tablet	PO	ACE inhibitor	q.d.	5mg, 10mg, 20mg, 40mg
captopril	Capoten	Tablet	PO	ACE inhibitor	b.i.d.–t.i.d.	12.5mg, 25mg, 50mg, 100mg
enalapril	Vasotec	Tablet, parenteral	PO, IV	ACE inhibitor	q.d.–b.i.d.	2.5mg, 5mg, 10mg, 20mg, 1.25mg/ml
fosinopril	Monopril	Tablet	PO	ACE inhibitor	q.d.	10mg, 20mg, 40mg
lisinopril	Prinivil, Zestril	Tablet	PO	ACE inhibitor	q.d.	2.5mg, 5mg, 10mg, 20mg, 40mg
moexipril	Univasc	Tablet	PO	ACE inhibitor	q.d.–b.i.d.	7.5mg, 15mg
quinapril	Accupril	Tablet	PO	ACE inhibitor	q.d.–b.i.d.	5mg, 10mg, 20mg, 40mg
ramipril	Altace	Capsule	PO	ACE inhibitor	q.d.	1.25mg, 2.5mg, 5mg, 10mg
trandolapril	Mavik	Tablet	PO	ACE inhibitor	q.d.	1mg, 2mg, 4mg
amiodarone	Cordarone, Pacerone	Tablet, parenteral	PO, IV	Antiarrhythmic	q.d.–b.i.d.	100mg, 200mg, 400mg, 50mg/ml
digoxin	Lanoxin	Tablet, capsule, liquid, parenteral	PO, IV, IM	Antiarrhythmic	q.d.	50mcg, 100mcg, 125mcg, 200mcg, 250mcg, 500mcg, 50mcg/ml, 100mcg/ml, 250mcg/ml
argatroban	Argatroban	Parenteral	IV	Anticoagulant	Infusion	100mg/ml
bivalirudin	Angiomax	Parenteral	IV	Anticoagulant	Infusion	12.5mg/ml
candesartan	Atacand	Tablet	PO	ARB	q.d.	4mg, 8mg, 16mg, 32mg
eprosartan	Teveten	Tablet	PO	ARB	q.d.	600mg
irbesartan	Avapro	Tablet	PO	ARB	q.d.	75mg, 150mg, 300mg
losartan	Cozaar	Tablet	PO	ARB	q.d.–b.i.d.	25mg, 50mg, 100mg
olmesartan	Benicar	Tablet	PO	ARB	q.d.	5mg, 20mg, 40mg
telmisartan	Micardis	Tablet	PO	ARB	q.d.	20mg, 40mg, 80mg
valsartan	Diovan	Tablet	PO	ARB	q.d.	40mg, 80mg, 160mg, 320mg
atenolol	Tenormin	Tablet, parenteral	PO, IV	Beta-blocker	q.d.	25mg, 50mg, 100mg, 5mg/10ml
bisoprolol	Zebeta	Tablet	PO	Beta-blocker	q.d.	2.5mg, 5mg
carvedilol	Coreg, Coreg CR	Tablet	PO	Beta-blocker	q.d.–b.i.d.	3.125mg, 6.25mg, 10mg, 12.5mg, 20mg, 25mg, 40mg, 80mg

(Continued)

Table 5-1. Common Cardiovascular Agents and Their Uses (Continued)

Generic Name	Brand Name	Dosage Form	Route	Common Use	Common Frequency	Common Strengths
labetalol	Normodyne, Trandate	Tablet, parenteral	PO, IV	Beta-blocker	b.i.d.	100mg, 200mg, 300mg, 5mg/ml
metoprolol succinate (ER)	Toprol XL	Tablet	PO	Beta-blocker	q.d.	50mg, 100mg, 200mg
metoprolol tartrate	Lopressor	Tablet, parenteral	PO, IV	Beta-blocker	b.i.d.	25mg, 50mg, 100mg, 1mg/ml
nadolol	Corgard	Tablet	PO	Beta-blocker	q.d.	20mg, 40mg, 80mg, 160mg
propranolol	Inderal, Inderal LA	Tablet, solution, parenteral	PO, IV	Beta-blocker	q.d.–q.i.d.	10mg, 20mg, 40mg, 60mg, 80mg, 120mg, 160mg, 1mg/ml, 4mg/ml, 8mg/ml
sotalol	Betapace	Tablet	PO	Beta-blocker	b.i.d.–t.i.d.	80mg, 120mg, 160mg, 240mg
amlodipine	Norvasc	Tablet	PO	Calcium channel blocker	q.d.	2.5mg, 5mg, 10mg
diltiazem	Cardizem, Cardizem SR, Cardizem CD, Dilacor XR, Diltia XT, Tiazac, Tiamate	Tablet, capsule, parenteral	PO, IV	Calcium channel blocker	q.d.–q.i.d.	30mg, 60mg, 90mg, 120mg, 180mg, 240mg, 300mg, 360mg, 5mg/ml
felodipine	Plendil	Tablet	PO	Calcium channel blocker	q.d.	2.5mg, 5mg, 10mg
nifedipine	Procardia, Procardia XL, Adalat, Adalat CC	Tablet, capsule	PO	Calcium channel blocker	q.d.	30mg, 60mg, 90mg
nisoldipine	Sular	Tablet	PO	Calcium channel blocker	q.d.	8.5mg, 10mg, 17mg, 20mg, 25.5mg, 30mg, 34mg, 40mg
verapamil	Isoptin, Isoptin SR, Calan, Calan SR, Verelan, Covera HS	Tablet, capsule	PO	Calcium channel blocker	q.d.–q.i.d.	40mg, 80mg, 120mg, 180mg, 240mg, 300mg, 360mg
bumetanide	Bumex	Tablet, parenteral	PO, IV	Diuretic	q.d.–b.i.d.	0.5mg, 1mg, 2mg, 0.25mg/ml
chlorthalidone	Hygroton	Tablet	PO	Diuretic	q.d.	25mg, 50mg, 100mg
furosemide	Lasix	Tablet, parenteral	PO, IV	Diuretic	q.d.–b.i.d.	20mg, 40mg, 50mg, 80mg, 10mg/ml
hydrochlorothiazide	HydroDIURIL	Tablet, capsule, parenteral	PO, IV	Diuretic	q.d.	12.5mg, 25mg, 50mg, 100mg, 50mg/5ml
indapamide	Lozol	Tablet	PO	Diuretic	q.d.	1.25mg, 2.5mg

(Continued)

Table 5-1. Common Cardiovascular Agents and Their Uses *(Continued)*

Generic Name	Brand Name	Dosage Form	Route	Common Use	Common Frequency	Common Strengths
metolazone	Mykrox, Zaroxolyn	Tablet	PO	Diuretic	q.d.	0.5mg, 2.5mg, 5mg, 10mg
spironolactone,	Aldactone	Tablet	PO	Diuretic	q.d.–b.i.d.	25mg, 50mg, 100mg
torsemide	Demadex	Tablet, parenteral	PO, IV	Diuretic	q.d.	5mg, 10mg, 20mg, 100mg, 10mg/ml
triamterene	Dyrenium	Capsule	PO	Diuretic	b.i.d.	50mg, 100mg
pentoxifylline	Trental	Tablet	PO	Improve blood flow in patients with circulation problems	t.i.d.	400mg
aliskiren	Tekturna	Tablet	PO	Miscellaneous antihypertensive	q.d.	150mg, 300mg
clonidine	Catapres	Tablet, patch, parenteral	PO, topically, IV	Miscellaneous antihypertensive	q.d.–q.i.d.	0.1mg, 0.2mg, 0.3mg, 100mcg/ml, 500mcg/ml
doxazosin	Cardura	Tablet	PO	Miscellaneous antihypertensive	q.d.	1mg, 2mg, 4mg, 8mg
hydralazine	Apresoline	Tablet, parenteral	PO, IV, IM	Miscellaneous antihypertensive	b.i.d.–q.i.d.	10mg, 25mg, 50mg, 100mg, 20mg/ml
prazosin	Minipress	Capsule	PO	Miscellaneous antihypertensive	q.d.–b.i.d.	1mg, 2mg, 5mg
terazosin	Hytrin	Tablet, capsule	PO	Miscellaneous antihypertensive	q.d.	1mg, 2mg, 5mg, 10mg
potassium supplements	K-Dur Tablets, Klor-Con, Slow-K Tablets, Micro-K Capsules, K-Lyte Effervescent	Tablet, capsule, liquid, powder, parenteral	PO, IV	Potassium supplement	q.d.	8mEq, 10mEq, 15mEq, 20mEq, 20mEq/15ml, 40mEq/15ml, 2mEq/ml,
enoxaparin	Lovenox	Parenteral	SQ	Prevent blood clot formation	q.d.–b.i.d.	30mg, 40mg, 60mg, 80mg, 100mg, 120mg, 150mg
heparin, unfractionated (UFH)	Hep-Lock	Parenteral	IV/SQ	Prevent blood clot formation	q.4–6h, continuous	10U/ml, 1000U/ml, 2000U/ml, 5000U/ml, 10,000U/ml, 12,500U/ml, 25,000U/ml,
warfarin	Coumadin	Tablet	PO	Prevent blood clot formation	q.d.	1mg, 2mg, 2.5mg, 3mg, 4mg, 5mg, 6mg, 7.5mg, 10mg,
ticlopidine	Ticlid	Tablet	PO	Prevent excessive blood clotting	b.i.d.	250mg

(Continued)

Table 5-1. Common Cardiovascular Agents and Their Uses *(Continued)*

Generic Name	Brand Name	Dosage Form	Route	Common Use	Common Frequency	Common Strengths
acetylsalicylic acid	Bayer Aspirin	Tablet, capsule, caplet, gelcap,	PO	Prevent heart attacks and strokes in at risk patients	q.d., q.4–6h	81mg, 325mg, 500mg, 650mg
clopidogrel	Plavix	Tablet	PO	Prevent heart attacks and strokes in at risk patients	q.d.	75mg
prasugrel	Effient	Tablet	PO	Prevent heart attacks and strokes in at risk patients	q.d.	5mg, 10mg
isosorbide dinitrate	Isordil	Tablet, capsule, sublingual tablet	PO, SL	Preventing and treating chest pain	t.i.d.	2.5mg, 5mg, 10mg, 20mg, 30mg, 40mg
isosorbide mononitrate	Imdur, Ismo/ Monoket	Tablet	PO	Preventing and treating chest pain	q.d.–b.i.d.	10mg, 20mg, 30mg, 60mg, 120mg
nitroglycerin	Nitro-Bid Ointment	Ointment	Topically	Preventing and treating chest pain	b.i.d.	2%
nitroglycerin	Nitro-Dur, Minitran	Patch	Topically	Preventing and treating chest pain	q.d.	0.1mg/hr, 0.2mg/hr, 0.4mg/hr, 0.6mg/hr
nitroglycerin	Nitrolingual	Spray	SL	Preventing and treating chest pain	PRN	0.4mg
sublingual nitroglycerin	Nitrostat/Nitroquick	Tablet	SL	Preventing and treating chest pain	PRN	0.3mg, 0.4mg, 0.6mg
atorvastatin	Lipitor	Tablet	PO	Reduce blood cholesterol	q.d.	10mg, 20mg, 40mg, 80mg
cholestyramine	Questran	Powder	PO	Reduce blood cholesterol	q.d.-b.i.d.	4g
ezetimibe	Zetia	Tablet	PO	Reduce blood cholesterol	q.d.	10mg
fenofibrate	TriCor, Lofibra, Triglide, Antara, Fenoglide	Tablet, capsule	PO	Reduce blood cholesterol	q.d.	40mg, 43mg, 48mg, 50mg, 54mg, 67mg, 120mg, 130mg, 134mg, 145mg, 150mg, 160mg

(Continued)

Table 5-1. Common Cardiovascular Agents and Their Uses (Continued)

Generic Name	Brand Name	Dosage Form	Route	Common Use	Common Frequency	Common Strengths
fluvastatin	Lescol, Lescol XL	Capsule	PO	Reduce blood cholesterol	q.d.	20mg, 40mg
gemfibrozil	Lopid	Tablet	PO	Reduce blood cholesterol	b.i.d.	600mg
lovastatin	Mevacor	Tablet	PO	Reduce blood cholesterol	q.d.	10mg, 20mg, 40mg
niacin	Niaspan	Tablet	PO	Reduce blood cholesterol	q.d.	500mg, 750mg, 1000mg
omega-3-Acid Ethyl Esters	Lovaza	Capsule	PO	Reduce blood cholesterol	q.d.–b.i.d.	1g
pitavastatin	Livalo	Tablet	PO	Reduce blood cholesterol	q.d.	1mg, 2mg, 4mg
pravastatin	Pravachol	Tablet	PO	Reduce blood cholesterol	q.d.	10mg, 20mg, 40mg, 80mg
rosuvastatin	Crestor	Tablet	PO	Reduce blood cholesterol	q.d.	5mg, 10mg, 20mg, 40mg
simvastatin	Zocor	Tablet	PO	Reduce blood cholesterol	q.d.	5mg, 10mg, 20mg, 40mg, 80mg
dipyridamole	Persantine	Tablet, parenteral	PO, IV	Reduce the risk of blood clots	q.i.d.	25mg, 50mg, 75mg, 5mg/ml
alteplase	Activase, t-PA	Parenteral	IV	Thrombolytic	PRN	50mg, 100mg
reteplase	Retavase	Parenteral	IV	Thrombolytic	PRN	10.4U (18.1mg)
streptokinase	Streptase,	Parenteral	IV	Thrombolytic	PRN	250,000U, 750,000U, 1,500,000U
tenecteplase	TNKase	Parenteral	IV	Thrombolytic	PRN	50mg
urokinase	Kinlytic	Parenteral	IV	Thrombolytic	PRN	250,000IU
nesiritide	Natrecor	Parenteral	IV	Treatment of heart failure	Infusion	1.5mg
dobutamine	Dobutamine	Parenteral	IV	Vasopressor	Continuous infusion	1mg/ml, 2mg/ml, 4mg/ml
abciximab	ReoPro	Parenteral	IV	Treatment of heart attack	Infusion	2mg/ml
eptifibatide	Integrilin	Parenteral	IV	Treatment of heart attack	Infusion	0.75mg/ml, 2mg/ml

Table 5-2. Miscellaneous Antihypertensive Combination Drugs

Brand Name	Generic Name	Common Use
Avalide	irbesartan/hydrochlorothiazide	Elevated blood pressure
Capozide	captopril/ hydrochlorothiazide	Elevated blood pressure
Dyazide, Maxzide	triamterene/ hydrochlorothiazide	Elevated blood pressure
Exforge HCT	amlodipine, valsartan, hydrochlorothiazide	Elevated blood pressure
Hyzaar	losartan/ hydrochlorothiazide	Elevated blood pressure
Lotrel	amlodipine/benazepril	Elevated blood pressure
Prinzide, Zestoretic	lisinopril/hydrochlorothiazide	Elevated blood pressure
Tenoretic	atenolol/chlorthalidone	Elevated blood pressure
Tribenzor	olmesartan, amlodipine, hydrochlorothiazide	Elevated blood pressure
Twynsta	telmisartan and amlodipine	Elevated blood pressure
Uniretic	moexipril/hydrochlorothiazide	Elevated blood pressure
Valturna	aliskiren and valsartan	Elevated blood pressure
Vaseretic	enalapril/ hydrochlorothiazide	Elevated blood pressure
Ziac	bisoprolol / hydrochlorothiazide	Elevated blood pressure
Caduet	amlodipine/atorvastatin	Elevated blood pressure, reduce blood lipids
Advicor	niacin/lovastatin	Reduce blood lipids
Vytorin	ezetimibe/simvastatin	Reduce blood lipids

Dosage Forms, Routes of Administration, and Usual Doses for Common Cardiovascular Medications

Most maintenance, or long-term, medications for high blood pressure come as tablets and capsules. It is not uncommon for tablets to be scored to allow for half-doses as well. Few liquid products are available, because most people who have high blood pressure are adults able to take oral medications. However, high blood pressure can also strike in the hospital, which is why several beta-blockers, ACE inhibitors, and other blood pressure medications are available parenterally as well.

Nitroglycerin is an example of a drug with several routes of administration. Sublingual (SL) tablets and sublingual sprays provide a very fast drug onset, allowing the drug to work immediately on existing pain from angina. They are not to be swallowed. Topical ointments, tablets, and patches provide longer-acting nitroglycerin capable of preventing pain from angina.

Some cardiovascular medications are used only in the inpatient setting. Infusion of these medications for one-time or short-term use may occur, particularly during treatment of cardiovascular issues. For instance, the treatment of a heart attack will likely involve several medications that are given parenterally.

Common Side Effects of Cardiovascular Medications

High blood pressure medications are obviously designed to decrease a person's blood pressure, so if the dose is too high, the patient may experience low blood pressure. This can be troublesome if it causes the patient to become lightheaded or dizzy or to pass out. Sometimes when a person sits up quickly after slouching or lying down, symptoms of a low blood pressure can become apparent. Also, immediately after increasing a dose, low blood pressure symptoms can occur, but they may go away after a few days.

Some cholesterol medications, the statins, can cause serious side effects. Although these side effects are rare, they can include muscle pain and liver damage. Practitioners will often require blood tests before prescribing these medications to confirm that a patient is not at a high risk for these effects.

Heparin, enoxaparin, warfarin, and other related drugs that decrease the risk for blood clots have the potential to increase the risk for bleeding. While in the hospital, a patient may be monitored closely if on heparin, and in the outpatient setting, a patient will likely receive regular blood work to monitor warfarin. A patient who is receiving too much medication may bruise easily or have trouble clotting after small cuts.

Terminology and Common Abbreviations Used with Cardiovascular Medications

See Table 2-1, page 13, for abbreviations.

What's in a name?

Table 5-3. Examples of USAN Stems for Cardiovascular Medications		
Stem	**Description**	**Example**
-arone	Antiarrhythmics	Amiodarone
-teplase	Tissue-type plasminogen activators	Alteplase
-azosin	Antihypertensives (prazosin type)	Doxazosin
-dralazine	Antihypertensives (hydrazine-phthalazines)	hydralazine
-sartan	Angiotensin II receptor antagonists	Irbesartan

Sample Prescription for Cardiovascular Medications

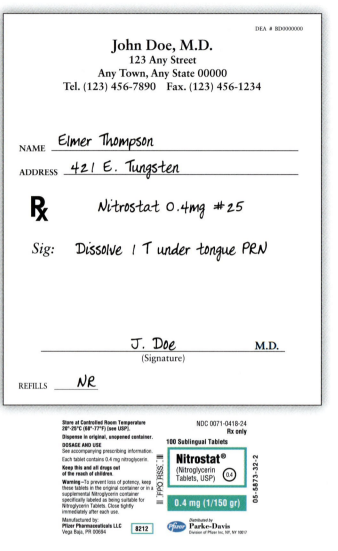

The above prescription should be interpreted as Nitrostat (nitroglycerin sublingual tablets) 0.4mg, dissolve one tablet under the tongue as needed. Dispense 25 tablets at a time with 5 refills.

Technician Tip

Sublingual nitroglycerin tablets must be dispensed in the original, amber glass container. Labeling requirements may be different on the smaller glass bottle than on a normal prescription vial and may vary by state. Check with your pharmacist if there is any confusion. ℞

Alternative Therapies for Cardiovascular Conditions

Patients who want to supplement their prescription medications or who want another option for their treatment may seek herbal supplements. Garlic is sometimes used to treat high blood pressure, as is folic acid and fish oil. Cholesterol may be treated with red yeast rice, garlic, fiber, and plant sterol and stanol esters. Often, these supplements are not as well tested as prescription medications and may even interact with prescription medications. Therefore, it is important for a patient to inform his or her pharmacist about any herbals, supplements, or over-the-counter medications that he or she is taking.

Lifestyle changes can also make a big difference in the treatment of cardiovascular conditions. Cholesterol may improve if saturated fat and cholesterol intake are decreased. Blood pressure may improve if a patient consumes less salt. Weight loss and increased physical activity can also have a significant impact on the treatment of both cholesterol and blood pressure.

Chapter Summary !

Cardiovascular medications can be used to treat several conditions, such as high blood pressure and high cholesterol. For inpatients, some cardiovascular drugs can be used to treat a heart attack or stroke. Chronic medications are given orally when possible, whereas some hospital medications are given intravenously. Some key categories of cardiovascular medications include:

℞ High blood pressure medications (antihypertensives), which include beta-blockers, calcium channel blockers, diuretics, ACE inhibitors, and ARBs

℞ High cholesterol medications, such as statins, bile acid resins, and fibrates

℞ Anticoagulants, such as warfarin and heparin

Several combination products also exist. Some combination products include two medications of the same class, such as two antihypertensives, whereas others have two or more purposes by combining medications from different classes.

STUDENT NAME _____

DATE _____ INSTRUCTOR'S NAME _____

ANATOMY, PHYSIOLOGY, AND PHARMACOLOGY QUESTIONS

Identify which of the following drugs can be used to treat high blood pressure or high cholesterol (circle one).

1. ACE inhibitors — High blood pressure — High cholesterol

2. Statins — High blood pressure — High cholesterol

3. Calcium channel blockers — High blood pressure — High cholesterol

4. Beta-blockers — High blood pressure — High cholesterol

5. Fibrates — High blood pressure — High cholesterol

Identify whether the following questions are true or false (circle one).

1. Arteries take blood away from the heart.
   TRUE   FALSE

2. High blood pressure is the same as hypertension.
   TRUE   FALSE

3. Thrombolytic agents are used to treat angina.
   TRUE   FALSE

4. Anticoagulants and thrombolytics have the same effect.
   TRUE   FALSE

5. Angiotensin II is the active form of angiotensin.
   TRUE   FALSE

MEDICATION QUESTIONS

Match the following brand-name products with their generic name.

1. _____ Tenormin

2. _____ Livalo

3. _____ K-Dur

4. _____ ReoPro

5. _____ Imdur

6. _____ Lanoxin

7. _____ Angiomax

8. _____ Lopid

A. potassium

B. bivalirudin

C. digoxin

D. gemfibrozil

E. isosorbide mononitrate

F. atenolol

G. abciximab

H. pitavastatin

9. _____ Altace

10. _____ Hytrin

11. _____ Micardis

12. _____ Questran

13. _____ Livalo

14. _____ Lotensin

15. _____ Cordarone

16. _____ Lovaza

A. terazosin

B. amiodarone

C. pitavastatin

D. ramipril

E. omega-3-acid ethyl esters

F. telmisartan

G. benazepril

H. cholestyramine

17. _____ Activase

18. _____ Apresoline

19. _____ Effient

20. _____ TriCor

21. _____ Corgard

22. _____ Demadex

23. _____ Lopressor

24. _____ Toprol XL

A. hydralazine

B. alteplase

C. nadolol

D. metoprolol tartrate

E. prasugrel

F. fenofibrate

G. metoprolol succinate

H. torsemide

25. _____ Procardia

26. _____ Lasix

27. _____ Avapro

28. _____ Pravachol

29. _____ Retavase

30. _____ Lovenox

31. _____ Persantine

32. _____ Betapace

A. irbesartan

B. enoxaparin

C. reteplase

D. furosemide

E. pravastatin

F. dipyridamole

G. sotalol

H. nifedipine

STUDENT NAME _____

DATE _____ INSTRUCTOR'S NAME _____

33. _____Norvasc

34. _____Aldactone

35. _____Niaspan

36. _____Coumadin

37. _____HydroDIURIL

38. _____Streptase

39. _____Nitrostat

40. _____Coreg

A. hydrochlorothiazide

B. amlodipine

C. niacin

D. carvedilol

E. spironolactone

F. sublingual nitroglycerin

G. streptokinase

H. warfarin

41. _____Vasotec

42. _____Inderal LA

43. _____Isordil

44. _____Cardizem

45. _____Bumex

46. _____Capoten

47. _____Calan

48. _____Cardura

A. diltiazem

B. enalapril

C. captopril

D. propranolol

E. verapamil

F. doxazosin

G. isosorbide dinitrate

H. bumetanide

Select the correct route of administration (circle one).

1. Nitrostat	Topical	Sublingual	Oral	Parenteral
2. dobutamine	Topical	Sublingual	Oral	Parenteral
3. Lescol	Topical	Sublingual	Oral	Parenteral
4. Lovenox	Topical	Sublingual	Oral	Parenteral
5. Trental	Topical	Sublingual	Oral	Parenteral
6. chlorthalidone	Topical	Sublingual	Oral	Parenteral
7. Nitro-Bid	Topical	Sublingual	Oral	Parenteral
8. Indapamide	Topical	Sublingual	Oral	Parenteral
9. Kinlytic	Topical	Sublingual	Oral	Parenteral
10. bisoprolol	Topical	Sublingual	Oral	Parenteral

Identify whether the following are available parenterally, orally, or both (circle one).

1.	clonidine	Parenteral	Oral	Both
2.	Crestor	Parenteral	Oral	Both
3.	Lovenox	Parenteral	Oral	Both
4.	Argatroban	Parenteral	Oral	Both
5.	fosinopril	Parenteral	Oral	Both
6.	Persantine	Parenteral	Oral	Both
7.	eptifibatide	Parenteral	Oral	Both
8.	heparin	Parenteral	Oral	Both
9.	TNKase	Parenteral	Oral	Both
10.	nesiritide	Parenteral	Oral	Both
11.	Lasix	Parenteral	Oral	Both
12.	quinapril	Parenteral	Oral	Both
13.	labetalol	Parenteral	Oral	Both
14.	prazosin	Parenteral	Oral	Both
15.	eprosartan	Parenteral	Oral	Both

Select the appropriate main use/drug class (circle one).

1.	bisoprolol	Beta-blocker	ACE inhibitor	ARB
2.	trandolapril	Beta-blocker	ACE inhibitor	ARB
3.	Benicar	Beta-blocker	ACE inhibitor	ARB
4.	moexipril	Beta-blocker	ACE inhibitor	ARB
5.	losartan	Beta-blocker	ACE inhibitor	ARB
6.	Sular	Diuretic	Calcium channel blocker	
7.	hydrochlorothiazide	Diuretic	Calcium channel blocker	
8.	Norvasc	Diuretic	Calcium channel blocker	
9.	nifedipine	Diuretic	Calcium channel blocker	
10.	Demadex	Diuretic	Calcium channel blocker	

STUDENT NAME _____

DATE _____ INSTRUCTOR'S NAME _____

Identify whether the following questions are true or false (circle one).

1. Metoprolol succinate is generic for Toprol XL, and metoprolol tartrate is generic for Lopressor.
   TRUE   FALSE

2. Nitrolingual is delivered intravenously.
   TRUE   FALSE

3. Cholestyramine is given in powder form.
   TRUE   FALSE

4. Streptokinase is considered a thrombolytic.
   TRUE   FALSE

5. Metolazone is delivered intravenously.
   TRUE   FALSE

6. Twynsta contains telmisartan and amlodipine.
   TRUE   FALSE

7. Zestoretic contains amlodipine and atorvastatin.
   TRUE   FALSE

8. Plavix is used to prevent heart attacks and strokes in at-risk patients.
   TRUE   FALSE

9. Lovastatin is used to prevent blood clot formation.
   TRUE   FALSE

10. Ticlid is delivered intravenously.
    TRUE   FALSE

Select a common strength for the following medications.

1. Bumex
   a. 0.1mg
   b. 0.2mg
   c. 0.5mg
   d. 0.8mg

2. Norvasc
   a. 5mg
   b. 50mg
   c. 500mg
   d. 5000mg

3. carvedilol
   a. 2.5mg
   b. 3.75mg
   c. 5mg
   d. 6.25mg

4. metoprolol succinate
   a. 10mg
   b. 50mg
   c. 500mg
   d. 1000mg

5. diltiazem
   a. 200mg
   b. 220mg
   c. 240mg
   d. 260mg

6. valsartan
   a. 20mg
   b. 50mg
   c. 80mg
   d. 100mg

7. Crestor
   a. 7.5mg
   b. 10mg
   c. 12.5mg
   d. 15mg

8. Lovenox
   a. 40mg
   b. 50mg
   c. 150mg
   d. 250mg

9. Plavix
   a. 10mg
   b. 25mg
   c. 50mg
   d. 75mg

10. Effient
    a. 10mg
    b. 25mg
    c. 50mg
    d. 75mg

11. lisinopril
    a. 7.5mg
    b. 25mg
    c. 40mg
    d. 50mg

12. Atacand
    a. 1mg
    b. 2mg
    c. 4mg
    d. 10mg

13. propranolol
    a. 40mg
    b. 50mg
    c. 60mg
    d. 70mg

14. Coumadin
    a. 100mcg
    b. 1mg
    c. 15mg
    d. 500mg

15. Zetia
    a. 5mg
    b. 10mg
    c. 15mg
    d. 20mg

STUDENT NAME _____

DATE _____ INSTRUCTOR'S NAME _____

Select the best available answer for the following questions.

1. Triamterene is considered a _____.

    a. beta-blocker
    b. diuretic
    c. calcium channel blocker
    d. ARB

2. Zestril and Prinivil are both brand names for _____.

    a. olmesartan
    b. lisinopril
    c. irbesartan
    d. fosinopril

3. Pravastatin is a drug that is used to _____.

    a. reduce blood pressure
    b. prevent blood clot formation
    c. supplement potassium
    d. reduce blood cholesterol

4. The generic name for Coreg is _____ and it is used as a _____.

    a. carvedilol, beta-blocker
    b. candesartan, ARB
    c. sotalol, beta-blocker
    d. nifedipine, CCB

5. Irbesartan is generic for _____.

    a. Avapro
    b. Ismo
    c. Atacand
    d. Isordil

6. Retavase is used as a _____.

    a. thrombolytic
    b. beta-blocker
    c. ARB
    d. anticoagulant.

7. Ziac contains _____.

    a. Olmesartan, amlodipine, and hydrochlorothiazide
    b. Irbesartan and hydrochlorothiazide
    c. Moexipril and hydrochlorothiazide
    d. Bisoprolol and hydrochlorothiazide

8. The proper route of administration of Plendil is _____ and its generic name is _____.

    a. PO, felodipine
    b. PO, verapamil
    c. IV, felodipine
    d. IV, verapamil

9. What do candesartan and olmesartan have in common? _____

    a. Both are ARBs
    b. Both are given IV
    c. Both are anticoagulants
    d. Both are available topically

10. Dyazide and Maxzide both contain _____.

    a. triamterene and hydrochlorothiazide
    b. moexipril and hydrochlorothiazide
    c. amlodipine and atorvastatin
    d. niacin and lovastatin

11. The generic name of Betapace is _____.

    a. atenolol
    b. prasugrel
    c. sotalol
    d. enoxaparin

12. Niacin is used to _____.

    a. prevent blood clot formation
    b. reduce blood cholesterol
    c. treat a heart attack
    d. prevent and treat chest pain

13. Avalide contains _____.

    a. amlodipine and atorvastatin
    b. irbesartan and hydrochlorothiazide
    c. amlodipine and benazepril
    d. aliskiren and valsartan

14. Atorvastatin is generic for _____.

    a. Lipitor
    b. Lescol
    c. Pravachol
    d. Zocor

15. Nitro-Dur is available as a _____.

    a. ointment
    b. tablet
    c. patch
    d. spray

STUDENT NAME _____

DATE _____ INSTRUCTOR'S NAME _____

16. Tekturna is the brand name of _____.

    a. alteplase
    b. lovenox
    c. losartan
    d. aliskiren

17. Vaseretic contains _____.

    a. atenolol and chlorthalidone
    b. triamterene and hydrochlorothiazide
    c. amlodipine and atorvastatin
    d. enalapril and hydrochlorothiazide

18. Zocor is available _____.

    a. parenterally
    b. topically
    c. orally
    d. sublingually

19. Eptifibatide is the generic name of _____.

    a. Tenormin
    b. Trandate
    c. Integrilin
    d. ReoPro

20. Zetia is used to _____.

    a. prevent heart attacks and strokes
    b. reduce blood cholesterol
    c. prevent and treat chest pain
    d. prevent blood clot formation

21. Diovan is a(n) _____.

    a. ACE inhibitor
    b. calcium channel blocker
    c. ARB
    d. beta-blocker

22. What do eptifibatide and abciximab have in common? _____

    e. Both may be used in the treatment of a heart attack
    f. Both are dosed q.i.d.
    g. Both are given p.o.
    h. Both treat high blood pressure

Match the following combination products with their ingredients.

1. _____ Capozide
2. _____ Tenoretic
3. _____ Advicor
4. _____ Exforge HCT
5. _____ Tenoretic
6. _____ Valturna
7. _____ Tribenzor
8. _____ Vytorin
9. _____ Lotrel
10. _____ Uniretic
11. _____ Hyzaar
12. _____ Prinzide

A. olmesartan, amlodipine, and hydrochlorothiazide
B. ezetimibe and simvastatin
C. atenolol and chlorthalidone
D. captopril and hydrochlorothiazide
E. amlodipine and benazepril
F. amlodipine, valsartan, and hydrochlorothiazide
G. atenolol and chlorthalidone
H. aliskiren and valsartan
I. moexipril and hydrochlorothiazide
J. niacin and lovastatin
K. lisinopril and hydrochlorothiazide
L. losartan and hydrochlorothiazide

DISCUSSION AND CRITICAL THINKING QUESTIONS

1. Why do many patients take more than one blood pressure medication?

_____

_____

_____

_____

_____

2. What lifestyle changes can people make to improve their blood pressure and cholesterol?

_____

_____

_____

_____

_____

_____

STUDENT NAME _____

DATE _____   INSTRUCTOR'S NAME _____

3. Will a patient's high blood pressure ever be cured by medication?

_____

_____

_____

_____

_____

4. Is it common to see prescriptions for hypertension medications dosed PRN? Why or why not?

_____

_____

_____

_____

_____

_____

5. Why might a patient prefer a nitroglycerin patch over a nitroglycerin tablet?

_____

_____

_____

_____

_____

_____

5. EXERCISES

SAMPLE PRESCRIPTIONS

DEA # BD0000000

John Doe, M.D.
123 Any Street
Any Town, Any State 00000
Tel. (123) 456-7890   Fax. (123) 456-1234

NAME Vincent Dorello

ADDRESS 4552 Thomasville

Rx Caduet 5mg/20mg #30

Sig: T 1 T PO QD

J. Doe M.D.
(Signature)

REFILLS RFx8

NDC 0069-2170-30
30 Tablets   Rx only
Caduet ®
(amlodipine besylate/
atorvastatin calcium)
5 mg/20 mg*
Distributed by
Pfizer **Pfizer Labs**
Division of Pfizer Inc, NY, NY 10017

1. What is the generic name for Caduet?

2. How would you translate the Sig code into plain English so that the patient could understand the directions for use?

3. How many refills are given on this prescription?

STUDENT NAME _____

DATE _____   INSTRUCTOR'S NAME _____

4. What common condition(s) does this medication treat?

_____

_____

DEA # BD0000000

John Doe, M.D.
123 Any Street
Any Town, Any State 00000
Tel. (123) 456-7890   Fax. (123) 456-1234

NAME _Shirley Martin_____

ADDRESS _1923 Clydesdale_____

Rx   Coumadin 1mg # 100

Sig: T 3 T PO QD on Mon, Wed,
            and Fri, at T 4 T PO QD
            on Tues, Thurs, Sat, and Sun

                    _J. Doe_____   M.D.
                     (Signature)

REFILLS _RFx 1____

---

1. What is the generic name for Coumadin?

_____

_____

2. How would you translate the Sig code into plain English so that the patient could understand the directions for use?

_____

_____

_____

_____

3. How many refills are given on this prescription?

_____

_____

_____

4. What other common strengths are available for Coumadin oral tablets?

_____

_____

_____

_____

5. What is a common use for this medication?

_____

_____

_____

_____

6. What is the days supply for this prescription?

_____

_____

_____

Technician Tip

Patients taking warfarin may switch between strengths on a regular basis and may have several warfarin prescriptions in their profile with refills remaining. If multiple warfarin prescriptions are on a patient's profile, it is important to ask which specific prescription he or she would like refilled. ℞

Diabetes and Thyroid Medications

6

KEY TERMS

Desiccated thyroid

Homeostasis

Hormones

Hyperthyroidism

Hypothyroidism

Insulin

LEARNING OBJECTIVES

After completing this chapter, the student will be able to:

1. Describe the basic anatomy and physiology of the endocrine system
2. Explain the therapeutic effects of common medications used to treat diseases of the endocrine system
3. List the brand and generic names of common medications used to treat diseases of the endocrine system
4. Identify available dosage forms for common endocrine medications
5. Identify routes of administration for common endocrine medications
6. Identify usual doses for common endocrine medications
7. List common side effects of frequently prescribed endocrine medications
8. Define medical terms commonly used when treating diseases of the endocrine system
9. List abbreviations for terms associated with use of medication therapy for common diseases affecting the endocrine system
10. Describe alternative therapies commonly used to treat diseases of the endocrine system

Basic Anatomy and Physiology of the Endocrine System

The endocrine system consists of 10 glands that work with the nervous system to maintain homeostasis. Homeostasis describes the ability of the body to maintain stable internal physiological balance, such as body temperature and the pH of blood, when environmental conditions change. Glands in the endocrine system secrete hormones into the bloodstream, and the hormones act on tissues, organs, and other glands. Hormones regulate a variety of processes in the body, including metabolic rate, production of enzymes, and the production of other hormones.

Glands of the endocrine system are shown in Figure 6-1 and include adrenal glands, hypothalamus, ovaries, pancreas, parathyroid glands, pineal gland, pituitary gland, testes, thymus gland, and thyroid gland.

The most common diseases associated with the endocrine system are thyroid disorders and diabetes. The most common thyroid disorders are hypothyroidism and hyperthyroidism. Hypothyroidism is a condition in which the thyroid gland produces too little of the thyroid hormones and in hyperthyroidism the thyroid gland produces too much of the thyroid hormones. Diabetes is associated with the pancreas and is usually characterized by inadequate secretion or utilization of insulin. Insulin is a hormone produced by the pancreas that regulates blood-sugar levels.

Knowing the following terms will be helpful as you learn about the medications used to treat conditions affecting the endocrine system.

Desiccated thyroid: thyroid glands that have been dried and powdered for therapeutic use

Homeostasis: the ability of the body to maintain stable internal physiological balance, such as body temperature and the pH of blood, when environmental conditions change

Hormones: chemicals that are secreted by glands into the bloodstream and function to regulate other processes in the body

Hypothyroidism: a condition in which the thyroid gland produces too little of the thyroid hormones

Hyperthyroidism: a condition in which the thyroid gland produces too much of the thyroid hormones

Insulin: a hormone produced by the pancreas that regulates blood sugar levels

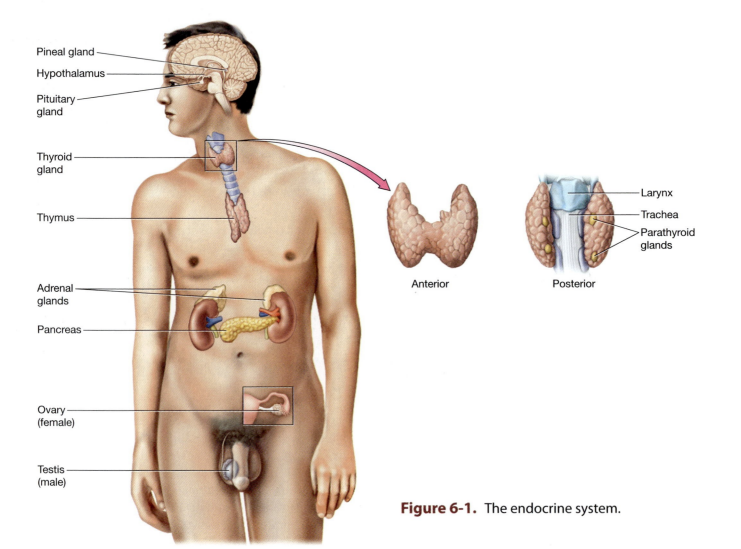

Pineal gland
Hypothalamus
Pituitary gland
Thyroid gland
Thymus
Adrenal glands
Pancreas
Ovary (female)
Testis (male)

Anterior

Larynx
Trachea
Parathyroid glands

Posterior

Figure 6-1. The endocrine system.

Primer on Pharmacologic Actions of Endocrine Agents

Endocrine medications can generally be thought of as drugs that perform the actions of hormones or that affect glands so that they produce more or less hormone. The most common endocrine medications are those used to treat hypothyroidism or diabetes. Disorders associated with reproductive hormones are also common, and drugs used to treat those disorders are covered in Chapter 11.

Thyroid Agents

Hypothyroidism can be treated by providing additional thyroid hormones. Thyroid hormones can be prescribed as desiccated thyroid, consisting of chemicals derived from an animal's thyroid gland, or synthetic thyroid hormones. There are two synthetic thyroid hormones: levothyroxine (Synthroid) and liothyronine (Cytomel). Additionally, liotrix (Thyrolar) is a mixture of levothyroxine and liothyronine.

Hyperthyroidism is a condition of too much thyroid hormone. Methimazole (Tapazole) is an example of a drug used to treat hyperthyroidism. Methimazole can also be prescribed for other conditions.

Antidiabetic Agents

Treatment for diabetes is aimed at controlling blood sugar. Treatment is individualized because the underlying disorder differs from patient to patient. Some patients require insulin injections. Other patients can take oral antidiabetic medications, and some patients are maintained on both insulin and oral antidiabetic medications.

Insulin is available in a number of forms. Aspart, detemir, glargine, glulisine, lispro, neutral protamine hagedorn (NPH), and regular (R) are common forms of insulin. The different forms of insulin vary by how rapidly they act and how often they must be administered.

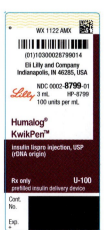

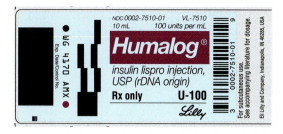

How is Humalog administered?

Blood sugar levels for some diabetic patients can be maintained by oral antidiabetic medications. It is important to know that oral antidiabetic medications work in different ways. There are four common classes of oral hypoglycemics: alpha-glucosidase inhibitors, biguanides, sulfonylureas, and thiazolidinediones. Acarbose (Precose) is an alpha-glucosidase inhibitor that lowers blood sugar by decreasing the absorption of carbohydrates from the gastrointestinal tract. Metformin (Glucophage) is a biguanide that lowers blood sugar by action on the liver. Glyburide (Micronase) is a sulfonylurea that lowers blood sugar by stimulating the pancreas to make more insulin. Pioglitazone (Actos) is a thiazolidinedione that lowers blood sugar by increasing sensitivity to insulin at the level of the cells.

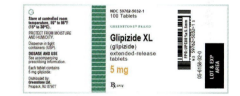

What is a common use for Glipizide XL?

Some common diabetes and thyroid agents and their uses are listed in Table 6-1.

Dosage Forms, Routes of Administration, and Usual Doses for Common Diabetes and Thyroid Medications

Thyroid medications are most often administered orally in the form of tablets. Because thyroid replacement medications are usually used for life, tablets

Table 6-1. Common Diabetes and Thyroid Agents and Their Uses

Generic Name	Brand Name	Dosage Form	Route	Common Use	Common Frequency	Common Strengths
NPH insulin	Humulin N	Parenteral	SQ	Intermediate-acting insulin	b.i.d.	U100
NPH insulin	Novolin N	Parenteral	SQ	Intermediate-acting insulin	b.i.d.	U100
insulin detemir	Levemir	Parenteral	SQ	Long-acting insulin	q.d.	U100
insulin glargine	Lantus	Parenteral	SQ	Long-acting insulin	q.d.	U100
insulin aspart	Humalog	Parenteral	SQ	Rapid-acting insulin	a.c.	U100
insulin glulisine	Apidra	Parenteral	SQ	Rapid-acting insulin	a.c.	U100
insulin lispro	NovoLog	Parenteral	SQ	Rapid-acting insulin	a.c.	U100
regular insulin	Humulin R	Parenteral	SQ, IV	Short-acting insulin	a.c.	U100
regular insulin	Novolin R	Parenteral	SQ, IV	Short-acting insulin	a.c.	U100
acarbose	Precose	Tablet	PO	Treatment of diabetes	t.i.d.	25mg, 50mg, 100mg
exenatide	Byetta	Parenteral	SQ	Treatment of diabetes	b.i.d.	5mcg, 10mcg
glimepiride	Amaryl	Tablet	PO	Treatment of diabetes	q.d.	1mg, 2mg, 4mg
glipizide	Glucotrol	Tablet	PO	Treatment of diabetes	q.d., b.i.d.	2.5mg, 5mg, 10mg
glyburide	DiaBeta, Micronase, Glynase	Tablet	PO	Treatment of diabetes	q.d., b.i.d.	1.25mg, 1.5mg, 2.5mg, 3mg, 5mg, 6mg
liraglutide	Victoza	Parenteral	SQ	Treatment of diabetes	q.d.	0.6mg, 1.2mg, 1.8mg
metformin	Glucophage	Tablet, liquid	PO	Treatment of diabetes	b.i.d.	500mg, 750mg, 850mg, 1000mg, 100mg/ml
metformin, glipizide	Metaglip	Tablet	PO	Treatment of diabetes	b.i.d.	2.5mg/250mg, 2.5mg/500mg, 5mg/500mg
metformin, glyburide	Glucovance	Tablet	PO	Treatment of diabetes	b.i.d.	1.25mg/250mg, 2.5mg/500mg, 5mg/500mg

(Continued)

Table 6-1. Common Diabetes and Thyroid Agents and Their Uses *(Continued)*

Generic Name	Brand Name	Dosage Form	Route	Common Use	Common Frequency	Common Strengths
miglitol	Glyset	Tablet	PO	Treatment of diabetes	t.i.d.	25mg, 50mg, 100mg
nateglinide	Starlix	Tablet	PO	Treatment of diabetes	t.i.d.	60mg, 120mg
pioglitazone	Actos	Tablet	PO	Treatment of diabetes	q.d.	15mg, 30mg, 45mg
pramlintide	Symlin	Parenteral	SQ	Treatment of diabetes	a.c.	60mcg
repaglinide	Prandin	Tablet	PO	Treatment of diabetes	t.i.d.	0.5mg, 1mg, 2mg
rosiglitazone	Avandia	Tablet	PO	Treatment of diabetes	q.d., b.i.d.	2mg, 4mg, 8mg
rosiglitazone, metformin	Avandamet	Tablet	PO	Treatment of diabetes	b.i.d.	1mg/500mg, 2mg/500mg, 4mg/500mg
saxagliptin	Onglyza	Tablet	PO	Treatment of diabetes	q.d.	2.5mg, 5mg
sitagliptin	Januvia	Tablet	PO	Treatment of diabetes	q.d.	25mg, 50mg, 100mg
sitagliptin and metformin	Janumet	Tablet	PO	Treatment of diabetes	b.i.d.	50mg/500mg, 50mg/1000mg
methimazole	Tapazole	Tablet	PO	Treatment of hyperthyroidism	t.i.d.	5mg, 10mg
propylthiouracil	Propylthiouracil	Tablet	PO	Treatment of hyperthyroidism	t.i.d.	50mg
levothyroxine	Levothroid, Levoxyl, Synthroid	Tablet, parenteral	PO, IV, IM	Treatment of hypothyroidism	q.d.	25mcg, 50mcg, 75mcg, 88mcg, 100mcg, 112mcg, 125mcg, 137mcg, 150mcg, 175mcg, 200mcg, 300mcg, 200mcg/10ml, 500mcg/10ml
liothyronine	Cytomel	Tablet, parenteral	PO, IV	Treatment of hypothyroidism	q.d.	5mcg, 25mcg, 50mcg
liotrix	Thyrolar	Tablet	PO	Treatment of hypothyroidism	q.d.	15mg, 30mg, 60mg, 120mg, 180mg
thyroid	Armour Thyroid	Tablet	PO	Treatment of hypothyroidism	q.d.	15mg, 30mg, 60mg, 90mg, 120mg, 180mg, 240mg, 300mg

allow for a simple method of daily administration. In the inpatient setting, thyroid medications may also be given parenterally should the patient be unable to take oral medication.

Most medications to treat diabetes are oral pills. Few liquids are available, because diabetes often affects adults who are able to take oral medication. The form of diabetes (Type I) that is more likely to affect small children is treated only with parenteral medications; oral medications rarely show benefit to Type I diabetes. Insulin is administered subcutaneously using either a vial and syringe or a pen device. Insulin pens require that a needle is attached to provide the injection.

Additionally, some insulins can be mixed in a syringe to reduce the number of times a person must inject in a day. For instance, if NPH insulin is to be given at the same time as regular insulin, the two can be mixed in a syringe and given together. Insulin is also produced in premixed ratios from the manufacturer to save the patient from having to do the mixing.

Common Side Effects of Diabetes and Thyroid Medications

Thyroid medications generally exhibit few side effects, but if the dosage is either too low or too high, side effects may become more pronounced. For instance, if the dose is too high, a patient may experience a fast heartbeat, fever, chest pain, excessive sweating, and weight loss. If the dose is too low, the patient may appear drowsy and lethargic and may gain weight.

Some medications used to treat diabetes may cause hypoglycemia, or low blood sugar, because they decrease a patient's blood sugar too much. Particularly if a patient does not eat regularly or is more physically active, hypoglycemia may present. Symptoms of hypoglycemia include weakness, fatigue, shakiness, and sweating.

Although many medications to treat diabetes, including insulin, may cause a patient to gain weight, exenatide and liraglutide may cause a person to lose weight. Metformin may cause an upset stomach and/or diarrhea. The dose of metformin may be started low and increased over several days, weeks, or even months in an attempt to limit such side effects.

Terminology and Common Abbreviations Used with Diabetes and Thyroid Medications

See Table 2-1, page 13, for abbreviations.

What's in a name?

Table 6-2. Examples of USAN Stems for Diabetes and Thyroid Medications		
Stem	**Description**	**Example**
-formin	Hypoglycemics (phenformin type)	Metformin
-glitazone	PPST agonists (thiazolidene derivatives)	Pioglitazone
-gliptin	Dipeptidyl aminopeptidase-IV inhibitors	Sitagliptin

Sample Prescription for Diabetes and Thyroid Medications

This prescription should be interpreted as Byetta (exenatide), 10mcg/0.4ml (2.4ml) pen. Inject 10mcg subcutaneously twice daily. One pen should be dispensed, which should last for 30 days.

DEA # BD0000000

John Doe, M.D.
123 Any Street
Any Town, Any State 00000
Tel. (123) 456-7890   Fax. (123) 456-1234

NAME _Tim Thomas_

ADDRESS _3134 W. Main_

℞   Byetta 10mcg #1 pen

Sig: Inject 10mcg SQ BID

J. Doe   M.D.
(Signature)

REFILLS _Rfx1_

Technician Tip

Byetta is an example of a medication that uses a prefilled, disposable pen. When getting ready to fill a prescription for an injectable medication, it may be worthwhile to ask the patient if he or she has enough needles or also needs a prescription for needles. ℞

Technician Tip

Many injectable medications will be found in the refrigerator in your pharmacy. However, just because they are stored in the refrigerator in the pharmacy does not always mean that the patient must refrigerate the medication. In fact, many insulins can be stored outside of the refrigerator for 30 days. Ask your pharmacist if you have any questions about storage requirements for medications. ℞

Alternative Therapies for Diabetes and Thyroid Conditions

Few alternative therapies exist for thyroid conditions. However, many lifestyle interventions and nondrug therapies exist for the treatment of diabetes. It is important to note that a patient should discuss any and all lifestyle interventions and alternative therapies with his or her physician before beginning additional treatment or discontinuing current treatment.

Health care practitioners may suggest several lifestyle interventions to treat diabetes, including increased physical activity, weight loss, and improved food choices. One popular food suggestion is to avoid simple sugars, such as those found in candy, ice cream, and regular soda. Alternatives such as diet soda may provide a sugar-free replacement, which may benefit the patient with diabetes.

Chapter Summary !

Thyroid medications are given to treat underproduction or overproduction of the thyroid gland. Although thyroid medications may be given for long periods of time, dose adjustments may be necessary. Both oral and parenteral medications are used to treat diabetes. Specific categories of diabetes medications include the following:

℞ Biguanides, such as metformin, which represent one of the more common oral medications for the treatment of diabetes

℞ Sulfonylureas, such as glipizide, which are another common category of oral medications that treat diabetes

℞ Insulin is one of the more common injectables; one person may take multiple kinds of insulin throughout the day at different times, and may even mix insulins

Patients with diabetes must also pay close attention to lifestyle modifications, such as food choices and changes in physical activity habits. When lifestyle modifications are combined with medicine, many patients can achieve good control of their diabetes.

STUDENT NAME _____

DATE _____   INSTRUCTOR'S NAME _____

ANATOMY, PHYSIOLOGY, AND PHARMACOLOGY QUESTIONS

Match the category of medication with its mechanism.

1. _____ Biguanide

2. _____ Alpha-glucosidase inhibitor

3. _____ Sulfonylurea

4. _____ Thiazolidinedione

A. Causes insulin production

B. Acts on liver

C. Reduces absorption

D. Improves insulin sensitivity

Identify whether the following questions are true or false (circle one).

1. Desiccated thyroid is not a synthetic product.

   TRUE   FALSE

2. Drugs used to treat hyperthyroidism often contain synthetic thyroid hormone.

   TRUE   FALSE

3. Insulin can be given orally.

   TRUE   FALSE

4. Antidiabetic agents are used to increase blood sugar.

   TRUE   FALSE

5. Insulin is a hormone.

   TRUE   FALSE

MEDICATION QUESTIONS

Match the following brand-name products with their generic name.

1. _____ Humalog

2. _____ DiaBeta

3. _____ Metaglip

4. _____ Precose

5. _____ Glucophage

6. _____ Levemir

7. _____ Avandamet

8. _____ Onglyza

A. rosiglitazone and metformin

B. insulin detemir

C. glyburide

D. glipizide and metformin

E. metformin

F. saxagliptin

G. acarbose

H. insulin aspart

6. EXERCISES

9. _____ Lantus
10. _____ Thyrolar
11. _____ Starlix
12. _____ Glucotrol
13. _____ Actos
14. _____ Januvia
15. _____ Amaryl
16. _____ Glucovance

A. glipizide
B. pioglitazone
C. glyburide and metformin
D. liotrix
E. nateglinide
F. sitagliptin
G. insulin glargine
H. glimepiride

17. _____ Glyset
18. _____ Micronase
19. _____ Apidra
20. _____ Prandin
21. _____ Cytomel
22. _____ Levoxyl
23. _____ Symlin
24. _____ Victoza

A. glyburide
B. insulin glulisine
C. liothyronine
D. liraglutide
E. miglitol
F. levothyroxine
G. repaglinide
H. pramlintide

Identify whether the following are available parenterally, orally, or both (circle one).

1.	levothyroxine	Parenteral	Oral	Both
2.	exenatide	Parenteral	Oral	Both
3.	Apidra	Parenteral	Oral	Both
4.	Avandia	Parenteral	Oral	Both
5.	Glyset	Parenteral	Oral	Both
6.	Symlin	Parenteral	Oral	Both
7.	Victoza	Parenteral	Oral	Both
8.	Tapazole	Parenteral	Oral	Both
9.	liothyronine	Parenteral	Oral	Both
10.	Armour Thyroid	Parenteral	Oral	Both

6. EXERCISES

STUDENT NAME _____

DATE _____ INSTRUCTOR'S NAME _____

Select the appropriate duration of action for each insulin product (circle one).

		Rapid	Short	Intermediate	Long
1.	Lantus	Rapid	Short	Intermediate	Long
2.	Novolin R	Rapid	Short	Intermediate	Long
3.	Humalog	Rapid	Short	Intermediate	Long
4.	Humulin N	Rapid	Short	Intermediate	Long
5.	Levemir	Rapid	Short	Intermediate	Long
6.	Novolin N	Rapid	Short	Intermediate	Long
7.	Apidra	Rapid	Short	Intermediate	Long
8.	Humulin R	Rapid	Short	Intermediate	Long
9.	NovoLog	Rapid	Short	Intermediate	Long
10.	insulin detemir	Rapid	Short	Intermediate	Long
11.	NPH Insulin	Rapid	Short	Intermediate	Long
12.	insulin lispro	Rapid	Short	Intermediate	Long

Identify whether the following questions are true or false (circle one).

1. Propylthiouracil is used for the treatment of hyperthyroidism.
   TRUE   FALSE

2. Armour Thyroid is used for the treatment of hypothyroidism.
   TRUE   FALSE

3. Miglitol is given subcutaneously.
   TRUE   FALSE

4. Janumet is a long-acting insulin.
   TRUE   FALSE

5. Apidra is used for the treatment of hypothyroidism.
   TRUE   FALSE

Select a common strength for the following medications.

1. Starlix
   a. 10mg
   b. 20mg
   c. 30mg
   d. 60mg

2. Glucotrol
   a. 2.5mg
   b. 7.5mg
   c. 15mg
   d. 30mg

3. metformin
   a. 100mg
   b. 250mg
   c. 500mg
   d. 1500mg

4. Avandia
   a. 1mg
   b. 2mg
   c. 5mg
   d. 10mg

5. Januvia
   a. 10mg
   b. 12.5mg
   c. 25mg
   d. 37.5mg

6. Armour Thyroid
   a. 20mg
   b. 30mg
   c. 40mg
   d. 50mg

7. Actos
   a. 5mg
   b. 10mg
   c. 15mg
   d. 20mg

8. Synthroid
   a. 1mcg
   b. 10mcg
   c. 100mcg
   d. 1mg

9. Byetta
   a. 1mcg
   b. 2mcg
   c. 4mcg
   d. 10mcg

10. Tapazole
    a. 2mg
    b. 10mg
    c. 50mg
    d. 500mg

Select the best available answer for the following questions.

1. The brand name for pramlintide is _____.

    a. Symlin
    b. Thyrolar
    c. Lantus
    d. Onglyza

2. Actos is used to treat _____.

    a. hypothyroidism
    b. hyperthyroidism
    c. diabetes
    d. none of the above

3. Identify the correct route of administration for glimepiride. _____

    a. IV
    b. IM
    c. Oral
    d. SQ

4. The medications contained in Avandamet are _____.

    a. rosiglitazone and metformin
    b. glipizide and metformin
    c. glyburide and metformin
    d. sitagliptin and metformin

5. The proper route(s) of administration of levothyroxine is/are _____ and it is used to treat _____.

    a. PO and IV, hypothyroidism
    b. IV, hypothyroidism
    c. PO, hyperthyroidism
    d. PO and IV, hyperthyroidism

6. The generic name of Amaryl is _____.

    a. glimepiride
    b. glyburide
    c. glipizide
    d. glulisine

7. The generic name for Onglyza is _____ and it is used to treat _____.

    a. saxagliptin, diabetes
    b. sitagliptin, diabetes
    c. nateglinide, hyperthyroidism
    d. repaglinide, hypothyroidism

8. The proper route of administration of Levemir is _____ and its generic name is _____.

   a. IV, regular insulin
   b. SQ, NPH insulin
   c. IV, insulin glargine
   d. SQ, insulin detemir

9. What do Synthroid and Cytomel have in common? _____

   a. Both treat diabetes.
   b. Both treat hypothyroidism.
   c. Both treat hyperthyroidism.
   d. Both are available subcutaneously.

10. Miglitol is a medication used to treat _____ and its appropriate route of administration is _____.

    a. diabetes, SQ
    b. diabetes, PO
    c. diabetes, IV
    d. hyperthyroidism, PO

STUDENT NAME _____

DATE _____ INSTRUCTOR'S NAME _____

DISCUSSION AND CRITICAL THINKING QUESTIONS

1. Why would a patient use two kinds of insulin at the same time?

_____

_____

_____

_____

_____

_____

2. How does your pharmacy handle the sale of insulin needles? Are there any special record-keeping requirements?

_____

_____

_____

_____

_____

3. Is it possible for people with diabetes to adjust their lifestyle to help treat the disease? If so, how?

_____

_____

_____

_____

_____

_____

_____

4. People with diabetes often use blood glucose meters to check their blood sugar. Why might it be helpful to know your blood glucose level if you have diabetes?

_____

_____

_____

_____

_____

5. If a patient experiences hypoglycemia from a diabetes medication, should he or she stop using the medication?

_____

_____

_____

_____

_____

_____

STUDENT NAME _____

DATE _____ INSTRUCTOR'S NAME _____

SAMPLE PRESCRIPTIONS

DEA # BD0000000

John Doe, M.D.
123 Any Street
Any Town, Any State 00000
Tel. (123) 456-7890   Fax. (123) 456-1234

NAME _Dorothy Fox_____

ADDRESS _583 Meadowbrook_____

Rx   Lantus # 1 vial

Sig: 20u QHS

_____J. Doe_____ M.D.
(Signature)

REFILLS _Rfx5_____

---

1. What is the generic name for Lantus?

   _____

   _____

2. What dosage form and route is appropriate for Lantus?

   _____

   _____

   _____

3. How would you translate the Sig code into plain English so that the patient could understand the directions for use?

_____

_____

_____

_____

4. How many refills are given on this prescription?

_____

_____

_____

5. How is this medication commonly categorized?

_____

_____

_____

_____

6. What is the days supply of this prescription?

_____

_____

_____

_____

STUDENT NAME _____

DATE _____ INSTRUCTOR'S NAME _____

DEA # BD0000000

John Doe, M.D.
123 Any Street
Any Town, Any State 00000
Tel. (123) 456-7890   Fax. (123) 456-1234

NAME _Teddy Frederick_____

ADDRESS _138 S. Front St._____

Rx   Glyset 50mg #90

Sig: T 1 T PO TID AC

_____ J. Doe   M.D.
                    (Signature)

REFILLS __NR____

---

1. What is the generic name for Glyset?

   _____

   _____

2. How would you translate the Sig code into plain English so that the patient could understand the directions for use?

   _____

   _____

   _____

3. How many refills are given on this prescription?

4. What other common strengths are available for Glyset oral tablets?

5. What condition is this medication used to treat?

6. What is the days supply of this prescription?

Technician Tip

Rapid- or short-acting insulins can sometimes be used with a "sliding scale," which may be abbreviated SS. In some instances, health care practitioners will want a patient to adjust his or her insulin on the basis of a recent blood-sugar reading. For instance, using the sliding scale, a blood glucose of 280 will require 3 units of Humulin R, and an insulin of 160 will require 1 unit of Humulin R. If the specific sliding scale is not indicated on the prescription, it is important to confirm that the patient received sliding scale instructions from his or her prescriber. If there is any confusion as to the directions, check with your pharmacist. ℞

STUDENT NAME _____

DATE _____ INSTRUCTOR'S NAME _____

DEA # BD0000000

John Doe, M.D.
123 Any Street
Any Town, Any State 00000
Tel. (123) 456-7890   Fax. (123) 456-1234

NAME *Marianne Hurt*

ADDRESS *917 Sparrow*

℞ *Humulin R # 1 vial*

Sig: *5u TID AC and per sliding scale*
SS: 150-200 = 1u, 200-250 =
2u, 250-300 = 3u,
300-350 = 4u, 350-400 = 5u,
> 400 = Call doctor

J. Doe   M.D.
(Signature)

REFILLS *RFx2*

NDC 0002-8215-01   HI-210
10 mL   100 units per mL

Humulin® R

REGULAR
insulin human injection,
USP (rDNA origin)
U-100   ◇
Lilly

---

1. What is the generic name for Humulin R?

   _____

   _____

2. How would you translate the Sig code into plain English so that the patient could understand the directions for use?

   _____

   _____

3. How many refills are given on this prescription?

   _____

   _____

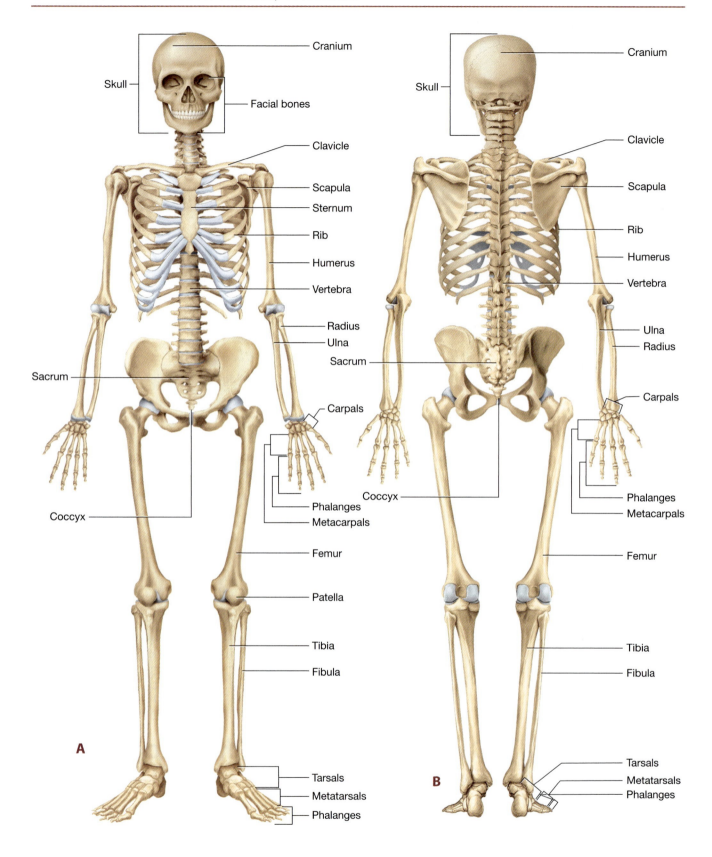

Figure 7-1. The human skeleton: (**A**) anterior view; (**B**) posterior view.

The muscular system consists of three main types of muscle in the body: skeletal muscle, smooth muscle, and cardiac muscle. Most skeletal muscle is attached to bones. See Figures 7-2 and 7-3 for anterior and posterior views of the muscular system in the body.

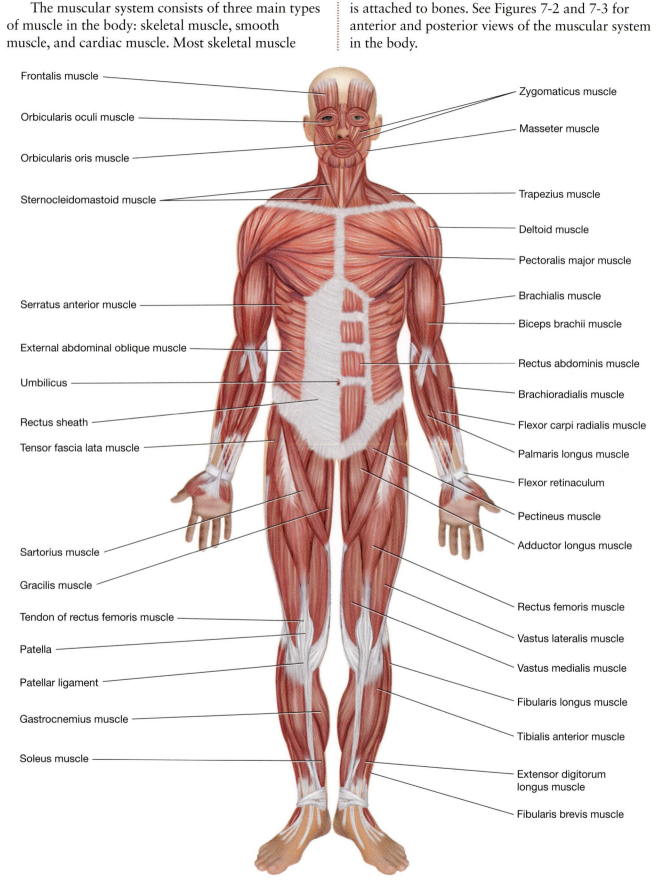

Frontalis muscle

Orbicularis oculi muscle

Orbicularis oris muscle

Sternocleidomastoid muscle

Serratus anterior muscle

External abdominal oblique muscle

Umbilicus

Rectus sheath

Tensor fascia lata muscle

Sartorius muscle

Gracilis muscle

Tendon of rectus femoris muscle

Patella

Patellar ligament

Gastrocnemius muscle

Soleus muscle

Zygomaticus muscle

Masseter muscle

Trapezius muscle

Deltoid muscle

Pectoralis major muscle

Brachialis muscle

Biceps brachii muscle

Rectus abdominis muscle

Brachioradialis muscle

Flexor carpi radialis muscle

Palmaris longus muscle

Flexor retinaculum

Pectineus muscle

Adductor longus muscle

Rectus femoris muscle

Vastus lateralis muscle

Vastus medialis muscle

Fibularis longus muscle

Tibialis anterior muscle

Extensor digitorum longus muscle

Fibularis brevis muscle

Figure 7-2. Muscles of the body, anterior view.

Parts shown include the frontalis muscle, orbicularis oculi muscle, orbicularis oris muscle, sternocleidomastoid muscle, serratus anterior muscle, external abdominal oblique muscle, umbilicus, rectus sheath, tensor fascia lata muscle, sartorius muscle, gracilis muscle, tendon of rectus femoris muscle, patella, patellar ligament, gastrocnemius muscle, soleus muscle, zygomaticus muscle, masseter muscle, trapezius

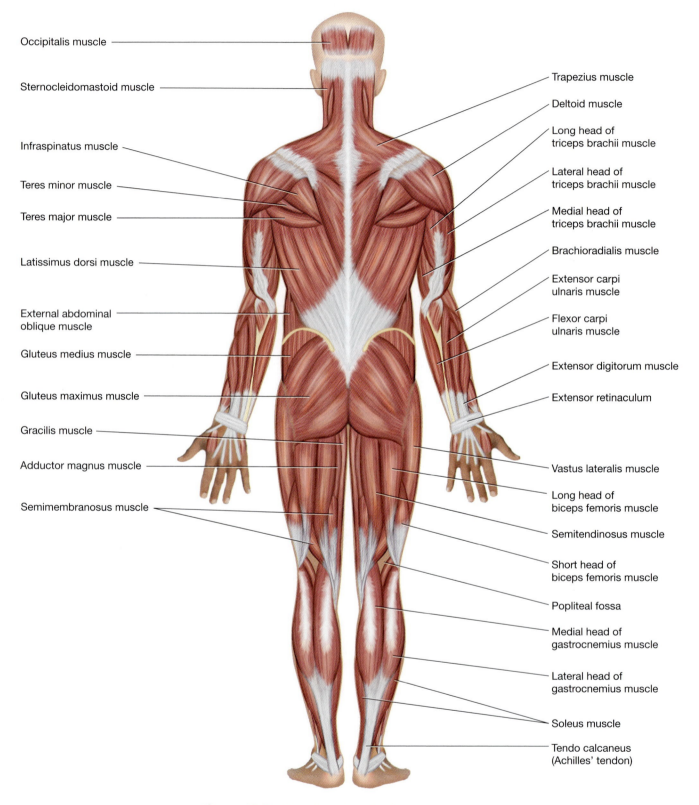

Occipitalis muscle

Sternocleidomastoid muscle

Infraspinatus muscle

Teres minor muscle

Teres major muscle

Latissimus dorsi muscle

External abdominal oblique muscle

Gluteus medius muscle

Gluteus maximus muscle

Gracilis muscle

Adductor magnus muscle

Semimembranosus muscle

Trapezius muscle

Deltoid muscle

Long head of triceps brachii muscle

Lateral head of triceps brachii muscle

Medial head of triceps brachii muscle

Brachioradialis muscle

Extensor carpi ulnaris muscle

Flexor carpi ulnaris muscle

Extensor digitorum muscle

Extensor retinaculum

Vastus lateralis muscle

Long head of biceps femoris muscle

Semitendinosus muscle

Short head of biceps femoris muscle

Popliteal fossa

Medial head of gastrocnemius muscle

Lateral head of gastrocnemius muscle

Soleus muscle

Tendo calcaneus (Achilles' tendon)

Figure 7-3. Muscles of the body, posterior view.

muscle, deltoid muscle, pectoralis major muscle, brachialis muscle, biceps brachii muscle, rectus abdominis muscle, brachioradialis muscle, flexor carpi radialis muscle, palmaris longus muscle, flexor retinaculum, pectineus muscle, adductor longus muscle, rectus femoris muscle, vastus lateralis muscle, vasus medialis muscle, fibularis tongus muscle, tibialis anterior muscle, extensor digitorum longus muscle, fibularis brevis muscle, occipitalis muscle, infraspinatus muscle, teres minor muscle, teres major muscle, latissimus dorsi muscle, gluteus medius muscle, gluteus maximus muscle, adductor magnus muscle, semimembranosus muscle, long head of triceps brachii muscle, medial head of triceps brachii muscle, extensor carpi ulnaris muscle, extensor retinaculum, vastus lateralis muscle, long head of biceps femoris muscle, semitendinosus muscle, short head of biceps femoris muscle, popliteal fossa, medial head of gastrocnemius muscle, lateral head of gastrocnemius muscle, soleus muscle, and tendo calcaneus (Achilles' tendon).

Knowing the following terms will be helpful as you learn about the medications used to treat conditions affecting the muscular and skeletal systems.

Analgesic: an agent that relieves pain

Bone: an organ of the skeleton

Cartilage: elastic tissue of the skeleton

Joint: point of contact between bones or cartilage

Narcotic: a drug derived from the opium plant that changes the way the body senses pain and thereby provides relief from pain

Osteoporosis: a condition in which bones become brittle, characterized by decreased bone mass and decreased bone density

Skeletal muscle: one of three types of muscle in the body that is commonly attached to bones

Skeleton: a collection of bones that provides structure and protection

Primer on Pharmacologic Actions of Musculoskeletal Agents

The most common musculoskeletal agents are analgesics. Other agents in this category include nonsteroidal anti-inflammatory agents (NSAIDs), skeletal muscle relaxants, and drugs to treat osteoporosis.

Analgesics are drugs used to treat pain. Morphine and codeine belong to a class of medications called narcotic analgesics. Narcotic analgesics are derived from the opium plant and change the way the body senses pain, providing relief from pain. NSAIDs also provide analgesic effects. They relieve pain by stopping the body's production of a substance that causes pain; this action also relieves fever and inflammation. These medications are non-narcotic and have more uses than narcotic analgesics. For example, they can be used for pain, tenderness, swelling, and stiffness caused by osteoarthritis and rheumatoid arthritis. Ibuprofen (Motrin) is an example of an NSAID.

Skeletal muscle relaxants work to relax muscles and relieve pain and discomfort caused by muscle injuries. Cyclobenzaprine (Flexeril) is an example of a skeletal muscle relaxant.

Osteoporosis is a condition in which the bones weaken and break easily. Drug therapy for osteoporosis is aimed at increasing the strength of the bones. Five types of drugs are commonly used to treat osteoporosis: bisphosphonates, estrogens, raloxifene, calcitonin, and synthetic parathyroid hormone. Bisphosphonates, such as alendronate (Fosamax), prevent bone breakdown and increase bone density. Estrogens, such as conjugated estrogens (Premarin), increase the density of bone. Raloxifene (Evista) is in a class of medications called selective estrogen receptor modulators (SERMs) and works by mimicking the effects of estrogen to increase bone density. Calcitonin (Miacalcin) works both to prevent bone breakdown and to increase bone density. Teriparatide (Forteo) is a form of synthetic parathyroid hormone that is also used to treat osteoporosis. It works by increasing the formation of new bone and by increasing the strength of existing bone.

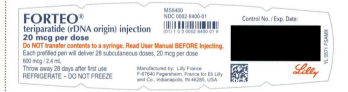

What is a common use for Forteo?

Some muscular and skeletal medications and their uses are listed in Table 7-1.

Table 7-1. Muscular and Skeletal Medications and Their Uses

Generic Name	Brand Name	Dosage Form	Route	Common Use	Common Frequency	Common Strengths
acetaminophen	Tylenol	Tablet, capsule, suppository, liquid	PO, rectally	For minor pain relief	q.4–8h	80mg, 120mg, 160mg, 325mg, 500mg, 650mg, 160mg/5ml, 80mg/0.8ml
acetaminophen and diphenhydramine	Tylenol PM	Caplet, liquid	PO	For minor pain relief and aid sleep	PRN	500mg/25mg, 500mg/25mg/15ml
acetaminophen, caffeine, pyrilamine	Midol	Caplet	PO	For minor pain relief associated with menstruation	q.6h	500mg/60mg/15mg
methyl salicylate and menthol	Bengay, Icy Hot	Balm, cream, stick, gel, patch	Topical	Temporary relief of minor aches and pains	q.d.–q.i.d.	29%/7.6%, 30%/10%
glucosamine and chondroitin	Osteo Bi-Flex	Caplet	PO	To reduce bone pain	t.i.d.	300mg/200mg
baclofen	Lioresal	Tablet	PO	To relax muscles	t.i.d.	10mg, 20mg
carisoprodol	Soma	Tablet	PO	To relax muscles	t.i.d.–q.i.d.	250mg, 350mg
cyclobenzaprine	Flexeril	Tablet, capsule	PO	To relax muscles	q.d.–t.i.d.	5mg, 7.5mg, 10mg, 15mg
metaxalone	Skelaxin	Tablet	PO	To relax muscles	t.i.d.–q.i.d.	800mg
methocarbamol	Robaxin	Tablet, parenteral	PO, IV, IM	To relax muscles	q.i.d., q.8h	500mg, 750mg, 100mg/ml
orphenadrine	Norflex	Tablet, parenteral	PO, IV, IM	To relax muscles	b.i.d.	100mg, 30mg/ml
tizanidine	Zanaflex	Tablet, capsule	PO	To relax muscles	q.6–8h	2mg, 4mg, 6mg
zoledronic acid	Zometa, Reclast	Parenteral	IV	To treat calcium issues of cancer, to treat osteoporosis	Once weekly, once yearly, every other year	4mg, 5mg
lidocaine	Lidoderm	Patch	Topical	To treat pain	Apply for 12 hours	5%
tramadol	Ultram	Tablet	PO	To treat pain	q.i.d.	50mg
tramadol, acetaminophen	Ultracet	Tablet	PO	To treat pain	q.i.d.	37.5mg/325mg
fentanyl	Actiq	Lozenge	PO	To treat pain (C–II)	q.4h	400mcg, 600mcg, 800mcg, 1200mcg, 1600mcg
fentanyl	Duragesic	Patch	Transder-mally	To treat pain (C–II)	q.72h	12.5mcg/hr, 25mcg/hr, 50mcg/hr, 75mcg/hr, 100mcg/hr
fentanyl	Sublimaze	Parenteral	IV/IM	To treat pain (C–II)	q.1-2h	50mcg/ml

(Continued)

Table 7-1. Muscular and Skeletal Medications and Their Uses *(Continued)*

Generic Name	Brand Name	Dosage Form	Route	Common Use	Common Frequency	Common Strengths
fentanyl	Onsolis	Buccal film	Bucally	To treat pain (C–II)	q.i.d.	200mcg, 400mcg, 600mcg, 800mcg, 1200mcg
fentanyl	Fentora	Buccal tablet	Bucally	To treat pain (C–II)	q.4.h.	100mcg, 200mcg, 400mcg, 600mcg, 800mcg
hydromorphone	Dilaudid	Tablet, capsule, liquid, parenteral	PO, IV, IM	To treat pain (C–II)	q.4–6h, q.24h	2mg, 4mg, 8mg, 12mg, 16mg, 24mg, 32mg, 1mg/ml, 2mg/ml, 4mg/ml, 10mg/ml
meperidine	Demerol	Tablet, liquid, parenteral	PO, IV, IM	To treat pain (C–II)	q.34h	50mg, 100mg, 50mg/5ml, 25mg/ml, 50mg/ml, 75mg/ml, 100mg/ml
methadone	Dolophine	Tablet, liquid, parenteral	PO, IV, IM	To treat pain (C–II)	q.3-4h	5mg, 10mg, 40mg, 5mg/5ml, 10mg/5ml, 10mg/ml
morphine	Roxanol	Tablet, solution, parenteral	PO, IV, IM	To treat pain, (C-II)	q.4h	15mg, 30mg, 10mg/5ml, 20mg/5ml, 1 mg/ml, 5mg/ml, 10mg/ml, 50mg/ml
morphine ER	MS Contin, Kadian, Avinza	Tablet, capsule	PO	To treat pain (C–II)	q.12–24h	15mg, 30mg, 50mg, 60mg, 90mg, 100mg, 120mg, 200mg
oxycodone	OxyIR, OxyFAST	Tablet, capsule, liquid	PO	To treat pain (C–II)	q.4–6h	5mg, 10mg, 15mg, 20mg, 30mg, 5mg/5ml
oxycodone ER	OxyContin	Tablet	PO	To treat pain (C–II)	q.12h	10mg, 15mg, 20mg, 30mg, 40mg, 60mg, 80mg
oxycodone, acetaminophen	Percocet, Tylox, Roxi-cet, Endocet	Tablet, liquid	PO	To treat pain (C–II)	q.4–6h	2.5mg/325mg, 5mg/325mg, 5mg/500mg, 7.5mg/325mg, 7.5mg/500mg, 10mg/325mg, 10mg/650mg
oxycodone, aspirin	Percodan	Tablet	PO	To treat pain (C–II)	q.4–6h	4.8355mg/325mg
codeine, acetaminophen	Tylenol with Codeine (#2)	Tablet, liquid	PO	To treat pain (C–III)	q.4–6h	15mg/300mg,
codeine, acetaminophen	Tylenol with Codeine (#3)	Tablet, liquid	PO	To treat pain (C–III)	q.4–6h	30mg/300mg,
codeine, acetaminophen	Tylenol with Codeine (#4)	Tablet, liquid	PO	To treat pain (C–III)	q.4–6h	60mg/300mg,

(Continued)

Table 7-1. Muscular and Skeletal Medications and Their Uses (Continued)

Generic Name	Brand Name	Dosage Form	Route	Common Use	Common Frequency	Common Strengths
methylprednisolone	Depo-Medrol, Medrol, Solu-Medrol	Tablet, parenteral	PO, IV, IM	Treatment of inflammation	q.d.–b.i.d.	2mg, 4mg, 8mg, 16mg, 32mg, 20mg/ml, 40mg/ml, 80mg/ml
prednisone	Deltasone, Orasone	Tablet, liquid	PO	Treatment of inflammation	q.d.–q.i.d.	2.5mg, 5mg, 10mg, 20mg, 50mg, 5mg/5ml
teriparatide	Forteo	Parenteral	SQ	Treatment of osteoporosis	q.d.	20mcg
adalimumab	Humira	Parenteral	SQ	Treatment of rheumatoid arthritis	Every two weeks	40mg
anakinra	Kineret	Parenteral	SQ	Treatment of rheumatoid arthritis	q.d.	100mg
azathioprine	Imuran	Tablet, parenteral	PO	Treatment of rheumatoid arthritis	q.d.–b.i.d.	25mg, 50mg, 75mg, 100mg
etanercept	Enbrel	Parenteral	SQ	Treatment of rheumatoid arthritis	1–2 times weekly	50mg/ml
hydroxychloroquine	Plaquenil	Tablet	PO	Treatment of rheumatoid arthritis	q.d.	200mg
infliximab	Remicade	Parenteral	IV	Treatment of rheumatoid arthritis	q.8 weeks	100mg
leflunomide	Arava	Tablet	PO	Treatment of rheumatoid arthritis	q.d.	10mg, 20mg
methotrexate	Rheumatrex	Tablet, parenteral	PO, IM	Treatment of rheumatoid arthritis	q.week	2.5mg, 5mg, 7.5mg, 10mg, 15mg, 25mg/ml
sulfasalazine	Azulfidine	Tablet	PO	Treatment of rheumatoid arthritis	b.i.d.	500mg

Technician Tip

Some injectable medications for rheumatoid arthritis may require refrigeration. When your pharmacy's supplier brings medications to the pharmacy, items requiring refrigeration should be promptly and appropriately stored. Your pharmacist may also want to counsel patients on proper storage of these medications at home. ℞

Dosage Forms, Routes of Administration, and Usual Doses for Common Muscular and Skeletal Medications

Many medications used for pain relief and muscle relaxation are given orally, either as capsules or tablets, to allow a person to maintain treatment at home. Liquids are also available should the patient be unable to take an oral pill. Parenteral formulations are also available, which allow for a faster onset of pain relief.

Fentanyl (Duragesic) is one example of a drug used transdermally in the form of a patch. Fentanyl can be a useful long-term pain-relief agent, and the patient can change the patch every three days rather than take a pill several times a day. Fentanyl lozenges (Actiq) are also useful for pain relief; they dissolve quickly in the mouth and are absorbed and begin working quickly.

Some medications used to treat rheumatoid arthritis must be injected to be effective. Although treatments for gout are commonly given by mouth, allopurinol may be injected.

Common Side Effects of Muscular and Skeletal Medications

Many medications that cause pain relief can also cause drowsiness, dizziness, or confusion. It is often recommended that a patient not drive or operate heavy machinery until after he or she is used to the effects of the pain reliever. Constipation is another common side effect with narcotic analgesics, and other treatments may be required to maintain regularity. Some other pain relievers, particularly NSAIDs, may cause an upset stomach, and even ulcers. Long-term users of NSAIDs may take additional medication to protect the stomach.

Some drugs used to treat osteoporosis can also cause stomach ulceration. For some osteoporosis medications, it is recommended that a patient take the tablet with a full glass of water and remain upright for 30 to 60 minutes. This may help to lessen the stomach pain and reduce the risk for a stomach ulcer.

Some medications used to treat rheumatoid arthritis can have gastrointestinal side effects, such as nausea and diarrhea. Some of the parenteral medications may make it easier for a person to acquire an infection; therefore, health care practitioners often observe the patient closely to determine whether he or she is getting sick while on the medication.

Terminology and Common Abbreviations Used with Muscular and Skeletal Medications

See Table 2-1, page 13, for abbreviations.

What's in a name?

Table 7-2. Examples of USAN Stems for Muscular and Skeletal Medications

Stem	Description	Example
-caine	Local anesthetics	lidocaine
-coxib	Cyclooxygenase-2 inhibitors	celecoxib
-ac	Anti-inflammatory agents (acetic acid derivatives)	diclofenac
-icam	Anti-inflammatory agents (isoxicam type)	meloxicam
-dronate	Calcium metabolism regulators	alendronate

Sample Prescription for Muscular and Skeletal Medications

This should be interpreted as tramadol/acetaminophen (sometimes called tramadol/APAP) 37.5mg/325mg, take one tablet by mouth every six hours as needed. Dispense 20 tablets. No refills.

DEA # BD0000000

John Doe, M.D.
123 Any Street
Any Town, Any State 00000
Tel. (123) 456-7890   Fax. (123) 456-1234

NAME _____ Rob Stark _____

ADDRESS _____ 1822 Lytham _____

Rx   Ultracet 37.5mg/325mg #20

Sig: T 1 T Q6H PRN.

_____ J. Doe _____ M.D.
(Signature)

REFILLS _____ NR _____

Alternative Therapies for Muscular and Skeletal Conditions

There are no commonly available herbal supplements that control pain as well as some of the agents listed in this chapter; therefore, many alternative therapies

Technician Tip

Tramadol and tramadol/APAP may not be controlled in your state, but it may have other reporting requirements. Your pharmacist may also want tramadol to be double counted, just as other controlled substances would be. Check with your pharmacist if you are unsure how tramadol is handled in your pharmacy. **Rx**

Technician Tip

Often times, medications have common suffixes that can give clues to their pharmacologic category or ingredients. When considering pain medications, many with brand names ending in "-cet" contain acetaminophen. This may be particularly helpful when trying to remember which combination products contain acetaminophen compared with other agents, such as Percocet/Percodan, Fioricet/Fiorinal, and Ultracet/Ultram. **Rx**

center on nondrug treatment options. For instance, many pharmacies carry heating pads that plug into the wall, can be heated in the microwave, or contain their own heating mechanism. Some are applied and stick to skin, such as in the lower back. Regardless of the method, it is important to follow a physician's orders closely when using a heating pad and not to let it get too close to a medicated patch, because the heat may change the rate at which the drug is absorbed into the body.

In some instances, pain is caused by a repeated motion or activity. Sometimes a physical or occupational therapist may be able to help a person find ways to work through an activity without it causing pain. Other times, a massage therapist may be able to help relieve muscle tension, which can also relieve pain.

Maintaining good hydration and reducing fat and alcohol intake may help to reduce the pain associated with gout, and thus patients being treated for this illness may report having a restricted diet. Assistive devices may be used to help with rheumatoid arthritis, because patients may have trouble with fine hand movements. Your pharmacy may sell items that allow a patient to grasp items, turn a door handle, or put on shoes, which may be helpful to a patient with advanced rheumatoid arthritis.

Chapter Summary !

One common musculoskeletal condition that is treated with medicine is pain. Whether the cause is arthritis, gout, a strain, or more serious damage, several pain control strategies are available.

℞ NSAIDs help to reduce inflammation and pain but may be irritating to the stomach

℞ Narcotics are often prescribed when pain control using NSAIDs or acetaminophen is insufficient. Special record-keeping and storage requirements may exist for narcotics in your pharmacy

℞ Rheumatoid arthritis may be specifically treated with its own set of medications. Some medications for rheumatoid arthritis may be injectable and have special storage requirements

Additionally, muscle relaxants can be used if pain is related to muscle problems. Prevention of other conditions such as osteoporosis is possible through oral medications taken chronically.

STUDENT NAME _____

DATE _____ INSTRUCTOR'S NAME _____

ANATOMY, PHYSIOLOGY, AND PHARMACOLOGY QUESTIONS

Identify whether the following categories of medications treat or prevent osteoporosis or whether they treat pain (circle one).

1. NSAID   Osteoporosis   Pain
2. SERM   Osteoporosis   Pain
3. Narcotic   Osteoporosis   Pain
4. Bisphosphonate   Osteoporosis   Pain
5. Synthetic parathyroid hormone   Osteoporosis   Pain

Identify whether the following questions are true or false (circle one).

1. Estrogens can be used to increase bone density.
   TRUE FALSE

2. NSAIDs are a type of narcotic.
   TRUE FALSE

3. A bone is considered an organ.
   TRUE FALSE

4. Osteoporosis is a condition in which bones become brittle.
   TRUE FALSE

5. Cartilage is one component of the skeleton.
   TRUE FALSE

MEDICATION QUESTIONS

Match the following brand-name products with their generic names.

1. _____ Boniva
2. _____ Mobic
3. _____ Ultram
4. _____ Decadron
5. _____ Kadian
6. _____ Clinoril
7. _____ Fortical
8. _____ Nuprin

A. dexamethasone
B. calcitonin
C. morphine ER
D. ibandronate
E. tramadol
F. sulindac
G. ibuprofen
H. meloxicam

3. How many refills are given on this prescription?

4. What is a common use for this medication?

Technician Tip

Ketorolac has a combined maximum 5-day duration of treatment. This duration is for both parenteral and oral use. Therefore, if a patient received three days of ketorolac in the hospital and is discharged with a prescription for dispensing in a community setting, only two days of ketorolac should be used. ℞

STUDENT NAME _____

DATE _____ INSTRUCTOR'S NAME _____

DEA # BD0000000

John Doe, M.D.
123 Any Street
Any Town, Any State 00000
Tel. (123) 456-7890   Fax. (123) 456-1234

NAME _____Alison Fronk_____

ADDRESS _____332 N. Oak St._____

Rx   Colcrys 0.6mg #30

Sig: T 2 T PO PRN gout pain.
            May take 1 T 1 hr after first
            dose. Max 1.8mg/day

_____J. Doe_____ M.D.
                (Signature)

REFILLS ___NR_____

1. What is the generic name for Colcrys?

   _____

   _____

2. How would you translate the Sig code into plain English so that the patient could understand the directions for use?

   _____

   _____

   _____

3. How many refills are given on this prescription?

4. What is a common use for this medication?

Technician Tip

Colchicine dosing recommendations have changed in recent years. New prescriptions that patients receive may not match the old prescriptions that they have on their profiles. If there is ever a question as to whether a dose is appropriate, check with your pharmacist. ℞

Nervous System Medications

8

KEY TERMS

Autonomic nervous system (ANS)

Brain

Central nervous system (CNS)

Cranial nerves

Homeostasis

Nerve impulses

Neuron

Peripheral nervous system (PNS)

Spinal cord

Spinal nerves

LEARNING OBJECTIVES

After completing this chapter, the student will be able to:

1. Describe the basic anatomy and physiology of the nervous system

2. Explain the therapeutic effects of common medications used to treat diseases of the nervous system

3. List the brand and generic names of common medications used to treat diseases of the nervous system

4. Identify available dosage forms for common nervous system medications

5. Identify routes of administration for common nervous system medications

6. Identify usual doses for common nervous system medications

7. List common side effects of frequently prescribed nervous system medications

8. Define medical terms commonly used when treating diseases of the nervous system

9. List abbreviations for terms associated with the use of medication therapy for common diseases affecting the nervous system

10. Describe alternative therapies commonly used to treat diseases of the nervous system

Basic Anatomy and Physiology of the Nervous System

The nervous system consists of the central nervous system (CNS) and the peripheral nervous system (PNS).

The CNS consists of the brain and spinal cord. Figures 8-1 and 8-2 show the brain and spinal cord.

The brain is the portion of the CNS contained within the skull. The spinal cord is continuous with the brain and is made of nerve cells called neurons, along with supporting structures. The CNS transmits nerve impulses for coordinating the activity of the entire nervous system.

The PNS lies outside the CNS and consists of nerves. The PNS mainly functions to connect the CNS to the arms, legs, and organs of the body. Cranial nerves originate from the brain, and spinal nerves originate from the spinal cord.

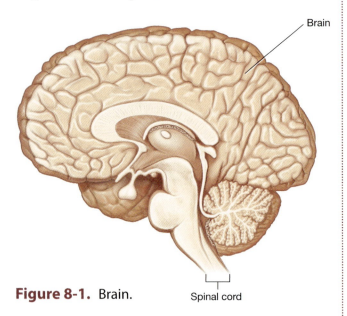

Figure 8-1. Brain.

Cranial nerves in Figure 8-3 include the following: olfactory nerve, oculomotor nerve, abducens nerve, trigeminal nerve, vestibulocochlear nerve, vagus nerve, hypoglossal nerve, spinal accessory nerve, glossopharyngeal nerve, facial nerve, trochlear nerve, and optic nerve. Spinal nerves in Figure 8-4 include the following: phrenic nerve, axillary nerve, musculocutaneous nerve, intercostal nerves, radial nerve, ulnar nerve, median nerve, lateral femoral cutaneous nerve, femoral nerve, pudendal nerve, saphenous nerve, sciatic nerve, common fibular nerve, tibial nerve, and sural nerve. Additionally, the autonomic nervous system (ANS) is a part of the PNS. The ANS functions to maintain homeostasis or relatively stable internal physiological conditions, such as body temperature and blood pH, even when the external environment changes. Regulation of the ANS is not subject to conscious control.

Knowing the following terms will be helpful as you learn about the medications used to treat conditions affecting the nervous system.

Autonomic nervous system (ANS): part of the PNS associated with maintaining homeostasis

Brain: the portion of the CNS contained within the skull

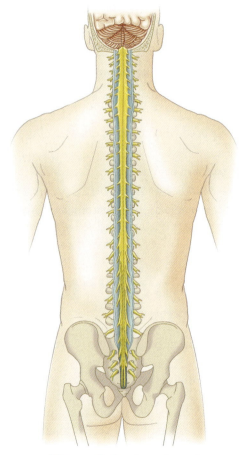

Figure 8-2. Spinal cord.

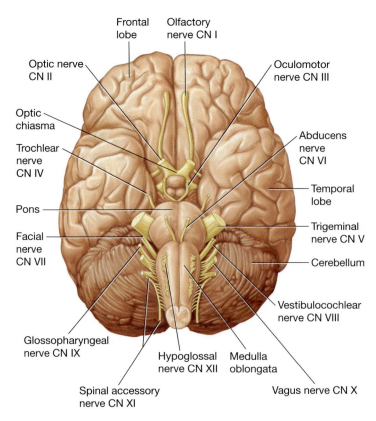

Figure 8-3. Cranial nerves.

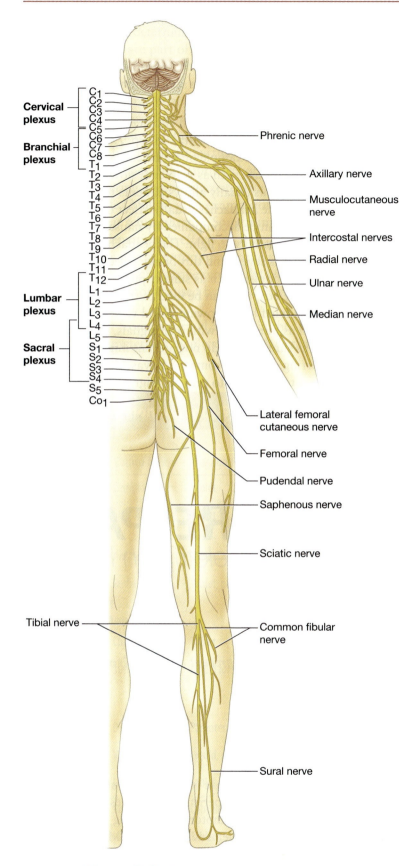

Figure 8-4. The spinal nerves.

Cervical plexus
Branchial plexus
Lumbar plexus
Sacral plexus

C1
C2
C3
C4
C5
C6
C7
C8
T1
T2
T3
T4
T5
T6
T7
T8
T9
T10
T11
T12
L1
L2
L3
L4
L5
S1
S2
S3
S4
S5
Co1

Phrenic nerve

Axillary nerve

Musculocutaneous nerve

Intercostal nerves

Radial nerve

Ulnar nerve

Median nerve

Lateral femoral cutaneous nerve

Femoral nerve

Pudendal nerve

Saphenous nerve

Sciatic nerve

Tibial nerve

Common fibular nerve

Sural nerve

Central nervous system (CNS): the brain and spinal cord

Cranial nerves: nerves in the PNS that originate in the brain

Homeostasis: relatively stable internal physiological conditions, such as body temperature and blood pH

Nerve impulses: transmission of sensations along nerves

Neuron: nerve cell

Peripheral nervous system (PNS): nerves outside of the CNS

Spinal cord: portion of the CNS that extends from the brain

Spinal nerves: nerves in the PNS that originate from the spinal cord

Primer on Pharmacologic Actions of Nervous System Agents

Nervous system agents are used to treat a wide variety of conditions affecting any aspect of the nervous system. The most common conditions treated by nervous system agents are attention deficit hyperactivity disorder (ADHD), Alzheimer's disease, anxiety disorders, bipolar disorder, depression, insomnia, migraine headaches, Parkinson's disease, schizophrenia, seizure disorders, and side effects of some antipsychotic medications

ADHD is a condition characterized by difficulty focusing, controlling actions, and remaining still or quiet. The disorder can occur in adults and children. Methylphenidate (Ritalin) is one medication used to treat ADHD, and it is also used to treat sleep disorders in some cases. Methylphenidate produces its effects by altering the amounts of some of the naturally occurring chemicals in the brain.

Alzheimer's disease is a disease of the brain that results in memory loss as well as loss of the ability to think and communicate. Donepezil (Aricept) is an example of a medication that improves mental function in patients with Alzheimer's disease and works by increasing the amount of a naturally occurring chemical in the brain called acetylcholine. It is important to know that medications such as donepezil do not cure Alzheimer's disease.

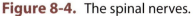

Table 8-1. Common Nervous System Agents and Their Uses *(Continued)*

Generic Name	Brand Name	Dosage Form	Route	Common Use	Common Frequency	Common Strengths
zolpidem	Ambien, Ambien CR	Tablet	PO	Sleep aid/insomnia (C-IV)	PRN	5mg, 6.25mg, 10mg, 12.5mg
nicotine	Commit	Lozenge	PO	Smoking cessation	PRN	2mg, 4mg
nicotine	NicoDerm CQ	Patch	Topically	Smoking cessation	q.d.	7mg, 14mg, 21mg
nicotine	Nicorette	Gum	PO	Smoking cessation	PRN	2mg, 4mg
rocuronium	Zemuron	Parenteral	IV	To facilitate intubation	PRN, infusion	10mg/ml
vecuronium	Norcuron	Parenteral	IV	To facilitate intubation	PRN, infusion	10mg, 20mg
atomoxetine	Strattera	Capsule	PO	To treat ADHD	q.d., b.i.d.	10mg, 18mg, 25mg, 30mg, 60mg, 80mg, 100mg
lisdexamfetamine	Vyvanse	Capsule	PO	To treat ADHD (C-II)	q.d.	20mg, 30mg, 40mg, 50mg, 70mg
dexmethyl-phenidate	Focalin, Focalin XR	Tablet, capsule	PO	To treat ADHD (C–II)	q.d., b.i.d.	2.5mg, 5mg, 10mg, 20mg
dextroamphet-amine	Adderall, Adderall XR	Tablet, capsule	PO	To treat ADHD (C–II)	q.d., b.i.d.	5mg, 7.5mg, 10mg, 12.5mg, 15mg, 20mg, 30mg
methylphenidate	Concerta	Tablet	PO	To treat ADHD (C–II)	q.d.	18mg, 27mg, 36mg, 54mg
methylphenidate	Daytrana	Patch	Transdermally	To treat ADHD (C–II)	q.d.	10mg/9hr, 15mg/9hr, 20mg/9hr, 30mg/9hr
methylphenidate	Metadate CD	Capsule	PO	To treat ADHD (C–II)	q.d.	10mg, 20mg, 30mg, 40mg, 50mg
methylphenidate	Ritalin, Ritalin LA, Ritalin SR	Tablet, capsule	PO	To treat ADHD (C–II)	q.d.–t.i.d.	5mg, 10mg, 20mg, 30mg, 40mg
modafinil	Provigil	Tablet	PO	To treat ADHD, fatigue (C–IV)	q.d.	100mg, 200mg
donepezil	Aricept	Tablet	PO	To treat Alzheimer's disease	q.d.	5mg, 10mg
galantamine	Razadyne	Tablet, capsule	PO	To treat Alzheimer's disease	q.d., b.i.d.	4mg, 8mg, 12mg, 16mg, 24mg
memantine	Namenda	Tablet	PO	To treat Alzheimer's disease	q.d., b.i.d.	5mg, 10mg
rivastigmine	Exelon	Capsule	PO	To treat Alzheimer's disease	b.i.d.	1.5mg, 3mg, 4.5mg, 6mg
tacrine	Cognex	Capsule	PO	To treat Alzheimer's disease	q.i.d.	10mg, 20mg, 30mg, 40mg

(Continued)

Table 8-1. Common Nervous System Agents and Their Uses *(Continued)*

Generic Name	Brand Name	Dosage Form	Route	Common Use	Common Frequency	Common Strengths
alprazolam	Xanax	Tablet, liquid	PO	To treat anxiety disorders (C-IV)	b.i.d.–t.i.d.	0.25mg, 0.5mg, 1mg, 2mg, 3mg, 1mg/ml
buspirone	BuSpar	Tablet	PO	To treat anxiety disorders	b.i.d.	5mg, 7.5mg, 10mg, 15mg, 30mg
chlordiazepoxide	Librium	Capsule, parenteral	PO, IV, IM	To treat anxiety disorders (C-IV)	t.i.d.–q.i.d.	5mg, 10mg, 25mg, 100mg
clonazepam	Klonopin	Tablet	PO	To treat anxiety disorders (C-IV)	t.i.d.	0.125mg, 0.25mg, 0.5mg, 1mg, 2mg
clorazepate	Tranxene	Tablet	PO	To treat anxiety disorders (C-IV)	b.i.d.–q.i.d.	3.75mg, 7.5mg, 11.25mg, 15mg, 22.5mg
diazepam	Valium	Tablet, liquid, parenteral, rectal gel	PO, IV, IM, rectally	To treat anxiety disorders (C-IV)	b.i.d.–q.i.d., q.3–4h	2mg, 5mg, 10mg, 20mg, 5mg/ml
lorazepam	Ativan	Tablet, parenteral	PO, IV	To treat anxiety disorders (C-IV)	b.i.d.–t.i.d.	0.5mg, 1mg, 2mg, 2mg/ml, 4mg/ml
meprobamate	Equanil	Tablet	PO	To treat anxiety disorders (C-IV)	b.i.d.–t.i.d.	200mg, 400mg
lithium	Eskalith, Lithobid	Tablet, capsule, liquid	PO	To treat bipolar disorder	b.i.d.–q.i.d.	150mg, 300mg, 450mg, 600mg, 300mg/5ml
amitriptyline	Elavil	Tablet	PO	To treat depression	q.d.	10mg, 25mg, 50mg, 75mg, 100mg, 150mg
bupropion	Wellbutrin, Budeprion	Tablet	PO	To treat depression	q.d.–b.i.d.	75mg, 100mg, 150mg, 200mg, 300mg
citalopram	Celexa	Tablet, liquid	PO	To treat depression	q.d.	10mg, 20mg, 40mg, 10mg/5ml
doxepin	Sinequan	Capsule, liquid	PO	To treat depression	b.i.d.–t.i.d., q.d.	10mg, 25mg, 50mg, 75mg, 100mg, 150mg, 10mg/ml
duloxetine	Cymbalta	Capsule	PO	To treat depression	q.d.	20mg, 30mg, 60mg
escitalopram	Lexapro	Tablet, liquid	PO	To treat depression	q.d.	5mg, 10mg, 20mg, 1mg/ml
fluoxetine	Prozac	Capsule	PO	To treat depression	q.d., weekly	10mg, 20mg, 40mg, 90mg
fluvoxamine	Luvox	Tablet	PO	To treat depression	q.d.	25mg, 50mg, 100mg
imipramine	Tofranil	Tablet, capsule	PO	To treat depression	q.d.	10mg, 25mg, 50mg, 75mg, 100mg, 125mg, 150mg

(Continued)

Table 8-1. Common Nervous System Agents and Their Uses *(Continued)*

Generic Name	Brand Name	Dosage Form	Route	Common Use	Common Frequency	Common Strengths
isocarboxazid	Marplan	Tablet	PO	To treat depression	b.i.d.–q.i.d.	10mg
mirtazapine	Remeron	Tablet	PO	To treat depression	q.d.	15mg, 30mg, 45mg
nefazodone	Serzone	Tablet	PO	To treat depression	b.i.d.	50mg, 100mg, 150mg, 200mg, 250mg
nortriptyline	Pamelor	Capsule	PO	To treat depression	q.d.	10mg, 25mg, 50mg, 75mg
paroxetine	Paxil, Paxil CR	Tablet	PO	To treat depression	q.d.	10mg, 12.5mg, 20mg, 25mg, 30mg, 37.5mg, 40mg,
phenelzine	Nardil	Tablet	PO	To treat depression	t.i.d.	15mg
sertraline	Zoloft	Tablet, liquid	PO	To treat depression	q.d.	25mg, 50mg, 100mg, 20mg/ml
trazodone	Desyrel	Tablet	PO	To treat depression	t.i.d., q.d.	50mg, 100mg, 150mg, 300mg
venlafaxine	Effexor	Tablet, capsule	PO	To treat depression	b.i.d.–t.i.d., q.d.	25mg, 37.5mg, 50mg, 75mg, 100mg, 150mg
acetaminophen, caffeine, butalbital	Esgic, Fioricet	Tablet	PO	To treat headaches	q.4h	325mg/40mg/50mg,
aspirin, caffeine, butalbital	Fiorinal	Tablet	PO	To treat headaches (C-III)	q.4h	325mg/40mg/50mg
acetaminophen, aspirin, caffeine (OTC)	Excedrin Migraine	Tablet, caplet, geltab	PO	To treat migraine headaches	q.4–6h	250mg/250mg/65mg
almotriptan	Axert	Tablet	PO	To treat migraine headaches	q.d., may repeat in 2 hours	6.25mg, 12.5mg
eletriptan	Relpax	Tablet	PO	To treat migraine headaches	q.d., may repeat in 2 hours	20mg, 40mg
frovatriptan	Frova	Tablet	PO	To treat migraine headaches	q.d., may repeat in 2 hours	2.5mg
naratriptan	Amerge	Tablet	PO	To treat migraine headaches	q.d., may repeat in 4 hours	1mg, 2.5mg
rizatriptan	Maxalt	Tablet	PO	To treat migraine headaches	q.d., may repeat in 2 hours	5mg, 10mg
sumatriptan	Imitrex	Tablet, nasal spray, parenteral	PO, IN, SQ	To treat migraine headaches	q.d., may repeat in 2 hours	5mg, 20mg, 25mg, 50mg, 100mg, 12mg/ml
zolmitriptan	Zomig	Tablet, nasal spray	PO, IN	To treat migraine headaches	q.d.	2.5mg, 5mg, 5mg/0.1ml

(Continued)

Table 8-1. Common Nervous System Agents and Their Uses (Continued)

Generic Name	Brand Name	Dosage Form	Route	Common Use	Common Frequency	Common Strengths
benztropine	Cogentin	Tablet, parenteral	PO, IV, IM	To treat Parkinson's disease	q.d.–b.i.d.	0.5mg, 1mg, 2mg, 1mg/ml
carbidopa, levodopa	Sinemet	Tablet	PO	To treat Parkinson's disease	b.i.d.–t.i.d.	10mg/100mg, 25mg/100mg, 25mg/250mg, 50mg/200mg
pramipexole	Mirapex	Tablet	PO	To treat Parkinson's disease	t.i.d.	0.125mg, 0.25mg, 0.5mg, 1mg, 1.5mg
ropinirole	Requip	Tablet	PO	To treat Parkinson's disease	t.i.d.	0.25mg, 0.5mg, 1mg, 2mg, 3mg, 4mg, 5mg
aripiprazole	Abilify	Tablet, liquid, parenteral	PO, IM	To treat schizophrenia	q.d.	2mg, 5mg, 10mg, 15mg, 20mg, 30mg, 1mg/ml, 7.5mg/ml
chlorpromazine	Thorazine	Tablet, liquid, parenteral, suppository	PO, IV, IM, rectally	To treat schizophrenia	q.4–6h	10mg, 25mg, 50mg, 100mg, 200mg, 25mg/ml, 100mg/ml
fluphenazine	Prolixin	Tablet, parenteral	PO, IM	To treat schizophrenia	q.6–8h	1mg, 2.5mg, 5mg, 10mg, 25mg/ml
haloperidol	Haldol	Tablet, liquid, parenteral	PO, IM	To treat schizophrenia	b.i.d.–t.i.d.	0.5mg, 1mg, 2mg, 5mg, 10mg, 20mg, 2mg/ml, 5mg/ml, 50mg/ml, 100mg/ml
olanzapine	Zyprexa	Tablet, parenteral	PO, IM	To treat schizophrenia	q.d.	2.5mg, 5mg, 7.5mg, 10mg, 15mg, 20mg
quetiapine	Seroquel	Tablet	PO	To treat schizophrenia	b.i.d.	25mg, 100mg, 200mg, 300mg
risperidone	Risperdal	Tablet, liquid, parenteral	PO, IM	To treat schizophrenia	q.d., b.i.d., q.2weeks	0.25mg, 0.5mg, 1mg, 2mg, 3mg, 4mg, 1mg/ml, 25mg, 37.5mg, 50mg
thioridazine	Mellaril	Tablet, liquid	PO	To treat schizophrenia	b.i.d.–q.i.d.	10mg, 15mg, 25mg, 50mg, 100mg, 150mg, 200mg, 30mg/ml
thiothixene	Navane	Capsule	PO	To treat schizophrenia	b.i.d.–t.i.d.	1mg, 2mg, 5mg, 10mg, 20mg
ziprasidone	Geodon	Capsule, parenteral	PO, IM	To treat schizophrenia	q.d., b.i.d.	20mg, 40mg, 60mg, 80mg
carbamazepine	Tegretol	Tablet, capsule, liquid	PO	To treat seizure disorders	b.i.d.–q.i.d.	100mg, 200mg, 300mg, 400mg, 100mg/5ml

(Continued)

Table 8-1. Common Nervous System Agents and Their Uses *(Continued)*

Generic Name	Brand Name	Dosage Form	Route	Common Use	Common Frequency	Common Strengths
divalproex sodium	Depakote	Tablet, capsule	PO	To treat seizure disorders	q.d.–q.i.d.	125mg, 250mg, 500mg, 100mg/ml
gabapentin	Neurontin	Tablet, capsule, liquid	PO	To treat seizure disorders	q.d.–t.i.d.	100mg, 300mg, 400mg, 600mg, 800mg, 250mg/5ml
lamotrigine	Lamictal	Tablet	PO	To treat seizure disorders	q.d.–b.i.d.	2mg, 5mg, 25mg, 100mg, 150mg, 200mg
levetiracetam	Keppra	Tablet, liquid	PO	To treat seizure disorders	b.i.d.	250mg, 500mg, 750mg, 100mg/ml
oxcarbazepine	Trileptal	Tablet, liquid	PO	To treat seizure disorders	b.i.d.	150mg, 300mg, 600mg, 300mg/5ml
phenytoin	Dilantin	Tablet, capsule, liquid, parenteral	PO, IV, IM	To treat seizure disorders	q.d.–t.i.d.	30mg, 50mg, 100mg, 200mg, 300mg, 50mg/ml
topiramate	Topamax	Tablet, capsule	PO	To treat seizure disorders	b.i.d.	15mg, 25mg, 50mg, 100mg, 20mg
valproic acid	Depakene	Capsule, liquid, parenteral	PO, IV	To treat seizure disorders	q.d.–q.i.d.	125mg, 250mg, 500mg, 100mg/ml, 250mg/5ml,
Pregabalin	Lyrica	Capsule	PO	To treat seizure disorders (C–V)	b.i.d.–t.i.d.	25mg, 50mg, 75mg, 100mg, 150mg, 200mg, 225mg, 300mg
Trihexyphenidyl	Artane	Tablet, liquid	PO	To treat side effects of some antipsychotic medications	q.d., t.i.d., q.i.d.	2mg, 5mg, 2mg/5ml

Dosage Forms, Routes of Administration, and Usual Doses for Common Nervous System Medications

Most medications listed in this chapter for nervous system conditions are used for long-term treatment. Therefore, oral pills are frequently used, particularly in conditions in which lifelong medication use may be required, such as depression or schizophrenia. Risperidone is an example of a medication that can also be given intramuscularly every two weeks. This may help if the patient does not want to take his or her medication, or has trouble remembering to take medication at the proper schedule. Liquid forms of

these medications are also available for a person who cannot take oral pills.

Nasal sprays can be used, particularly for migraine headaches, because this is also a way to get the medication to work quickly. Some people with migraines have tremendous pain when trying to eat or take anything by mouth; therefore, a nasal spray, or even a subcutaneous injection, may be a better route of administration than an oral tablet.

Medications used to help a patient sleep are given by mouth, allowing the patient the flexibility to decide when he or she needs help sleeping. Additionally, medications to help treat addictions are most often given by mouth so that the patient can self-treat from home. For example, varenicline may be taken for several months to help a patient quit smoking, and the medication being in tablet form allows the patient to maintain treatment without seeing a health care professional on a frequent basis.

Common Side Effects of Nervous System Medications

Antidepressants unfortunately have several side effects that are concerning to patients. However, not all side effects are common, and many people are able to take antidepressants for long periods with few issues. Side effects may include fatigue, headache, and sexual dysfunction. An increased risk for suicide may be seen, particularly in the first month of use. Interestingly, side effects are not always predictable. For instance, some people experience insomnia, whereas others experience somnolence; while some people exhibit weight gain, but others experience anorexia.

Many antianxiety medications may cause drowsiness, sedation, and confusion. Medications that treat insomnia may also cause someone to have difficulty waking in the morning, particularly if their schedule did not permit a full night's sleep. When taking medications from either class, it is important for patients not to operate heavy machinery or attempt to drive, at least until they understand how the medication will affect them.

Medications used to treat schizophrenia may also show somnolence as a major side effect. Weight gain, dizziness, headache, insomnia, and constipation may occur as well. Treatment for seizures may also involve dizziness, somnolence, headache, and weight gain.

Alzheimer's medications differ in their side-effect profile from some other medications listed in this section. Insomnia, agitation, and anxiety can be seen. Nausea, constipation, upset stomach, and headache are also noted.

The most common side effects associated with sleep aids is drowsiness, particularly if a patient chooses to sleep for less than 7 to 8 hours. Medications used to aid in the treatment of addictions may also cause drowsiness but could also cause insomnia or anxiety. Furthermore, vivid dreams may be experienced when a person is taking some addiction medications, particularly varenicline.

Terminology and Common Abbreviations Used with Nervous System Medications

See Table 2-1, page 13, for abbreviations.

What's in a name?

Table 8-2. Examples of USAN Stems for Nervous System Medications

Stem	Description	Example
-nicline	Nicotinic acetylcholine receptor partial agonists/agonists	varenicline
-flurane	General inhalation anesthetics	desflurane
-plon	Non-benzodiazepine anxiolytics, sedatives, hypnotics	zaleplon
-pidem	Hypnotics/sedatives (zolpidem type)	zolpidem
-pezil	Acetylcholinesterase inhibitors used in the treatment of Alzheimer's disease	donepezil

Sample Prescription for Nervous System Medications

This prescription should be interpreted as Ritalin (methylphenidate) 5mg tablets, take one tablet by mouth 30 minutes before breakfast and one tablet by mouth 30 minutes before lunch. Dispense 60 tablets. No refills.

DEA # BD0000000

John Doe, M.D.
123 Any Street
Any Town, Any State 00000
Tel. (123) 456-7890   Fax. (123) 456-1234

NAME ____ Donovan McCreary

ADDRESS ____ 8247 Dublin Ct.

℞   Ritalin 5mg #60 (sixty)

Sig: T 1 TPO 30 min before breakfast, lunch

_____ J. Doe _____ M.D.
(Signature)

REFILL ____ NR

Technician Tip

A physician's DEA number would be required on this prescription, because it is a C-II medication. Other record-keeping requirements will likely be required at your pharmacy, and C-II medications will probably be stored in a different location from non-C-II medications. Check with your pharmacist if you are unsure about requirements surrounding C-II medications in your pharmacy. ℞

Alternative Therapies for Nervous System Conditions

Self-management may be possible for insomnia. In some people, relaxation techniques, reducing or eliminating caffeine intake (particularly near the bedtime hours), and limiting excess light (e.g., computer use, watching television) and sound at bedtime can help encourage healthy sleep patterns. Melatonin is one dietary supplement that may be recommended to encourage healthy sleep patterns as well. As always, a patient should check with his or her physician before taking dietary supplements.

Many alternative therapies revolve around counseling with a trained professional, particularly depression, schizophrenia, and bipolar disorder. Support groups and counseling may supplement the medication used to treat addictions.

Chapter Summary !

Many central nervous system (CNS) conditions exist, and many medications are available to treat CNS conditions.

℞ Antidepressants come in several forms, each with its own specific niche and purpose

℞ Antipsychotic drugs can be used to treat conditions such as schizophrenia

℞ Additional medications are available to treat seizures and Alzheimer's disease, among other conditions

℞ ADHD is often treated with stimulants, which are Schedule II drugs. These medications will often have different record-keeping and storage requirements in your pharmacy

℞ Specific migraine headache medications exist that work quickly; some migraine medications can be given intranasally or may even be injected for fast relief

For some conditions, CNS medications will need to be taken for long periods of time to provide adequate control, because many CNS issues are not curable. In other instances, such as for migraine headaches or sleep aids, it may be appropriate to see medications dosed on an as-needed basis.

STUDENT NAME _____

DATE _____ INSTRUCTOR'S NAME _____

ANATOMY, PHYSIOLOGY, AND PHARMACOLOGY QUESTIONS

Identify whether the following are a part of the CNS or PNS (circle one).

1. Spinal nerves   CNS   PNS
2. Spinal cord   CNS   PNS
3. Brain   CNS   PNS
4. ANS   CNS   PNS
5. Cranial nerves   CNS   PNS

Identify whether the following questions are true or false (circle one).

1. Alzheimer's disease and ADHD are treated using the same categories of medications.
   TRUE   FALSE

2. Benzodiazepines and stimulants produce opposite effects.
   TRUE   FALSE

3. Selective serotonin receptor agonists prevent migraine headaches.
   TRUE   FALSE

4. Antipsychotic drugs can be used to help treat schizophrenia.
   TRUE   FALSE

5. Antiepileptic medications help to treat Parkinson's disease.
   TRUE   FALSE

MEDICATION QUESTIONS

Match the following brand-name products with their generic names.

1. _____ Aricept
2. _____ Haldol
3. _____ BuSpar
4. _____ Risperdal
5. _____ Cognex
6. _____ Mirapex
7. _____ Lyrica
8. _____ Daytrana

A.   donepezil
B.   tacrine
C.   haloperidol
D.   methylphenidate
E.   pregabalin
F.   pramipexole
G.   buspirone
H.   risperidone

8. EXERCISES

9. _____ Librium	A. topiramate
10. _____ Paxil	B. clonazepam
11. _____ Lexapro	C. trazodone
12. _____ Zoloft	D. sertraline
13. _____ Klonopin	E. alprazolam
14. _____ Topamax	F. paroxetine
15. _____ Xanax	G. chlordiazepoxide
16. _____ Desyrel	H. escitalopram

17. _____ Prozac	A. midazolam
18. _____ Antabuse	B. fluoxetine
19. _____ Sonata	C. almotriptan
20. _____ Versed	D. lisdexamfetamine
21. _____ Frova	E. disulfiram
22. _____ Axert	F. frovatriptan
23. _____ Vyvanse	G. zaleplon
24. _____ Ambien CR	H. zolpidem

25. _____ Zemuron	A. varenicline
26. _____ Geodon	B. dextroamphetamine
27. _____ Namenda	C. rocuronium
28. _____ Razadyne	D. ziprasidone
29. _____ Lunesta	E. methylphenidate
30. _____ Chantix	F. memantine
31. _____ Metadate CD	G. galantamine
32. _____ Adderall XR	H. eszopiclone

STUDENT NAME _____

DATE _____ INSTRUCTOR'S NAME _____

33. _____ Seroquel

34. _____ Cogentin

35. _____ Tofranil

36. _____ Keppra

37. _____ Dilantin

38. _____ Ritalin LA

39. _____ Zyprexa

40. _____ Requip

A. methylphenidate

B. ropinirole

C. benztropine

D. quetiapine

E. levetiracetam

F. imipramine

G. phenytoin

H. olanzapine

41. _____ Wellbutrin

42. _____ Imitrex

43. _____ Zomig

44. _____ Provigil

45. _____ Abilify

46. _____ Sinemet

47. _____ Strattera

48. _____ Depakote

A. aripiprazole

B. sumatriptan

C. carbidopa and levodopa

D. bupropion

E. divalproex sodium

F. modafinil

G. zolmitriptan

H. atomoxetine

49. _____ Amerge

50. _____ Tegretol

51. _____ Fioricet

52. _____ Depakene

53. _____ Fiorinal

54. _____ Ambien

55. _____ Halcion

56. _____ Ativan

A. zolpidem

B. naratriptan

C. triazolam

D. valproic acid

E. acetaminophen, caffeine, butalbital

F. lorazepam

G. aspirin, caffeine, butalbital

H. carbamazepine

57. _____ Tranxene

58. _____ Sinequan

59. _____ Lamictal

60. _____ ReVia

61. _____ Maxalt

62. _____ Trileptal

63. _____ Serzone

64. _____ Remeron

A. lamotrigine

B. mirtazapine

C. oxcarbazepine

D. rizatriptan

E. naltrexone

F. doxepin

G. nefazodone

H. clorazepate

Select a common and appropriate frequency of administration (circle one).

		q.d.	b.i.d.	t.i.d.
1.	Zyprexa	q.d.	b.i.d.	t.i.d.
2.	Trileptal	q.d.	b.i.d.	t.i.d.
3.	Topamax	q.d.	b.i.d.	t.i.d.
4.	amitriptyline	q.d.	b.i.d.	t.i.d.
5.	sertraline	q.d.	b.i.d.	t.i.d.
6.	Vyvanse	q.d.	b.i.d.	t.i.d.
7.	Requip	q.d.	b.i.d.	t.i.d.
8.	Seroquel	q.d.	b.i.d.	t.i.d.
9.	pramipexole	q.d.	b.i.d.	t.i.d.
10.	citalopram	q.d.	b.i.d.	t.i.d.

Select the correct route of administration (circle one).

1.	Xanax	Transdermally	PO	IV
2.	vecuronium	Transdermally	PO	IV
3.	Lexapro	Transdermally	PO	IV
4.	Daytrana	Transdermally	PO	IV
5.	trihexyphenidyl	Transdermally	PO	IV
6.	rocuronium	Transdermally	PO	IV
7.	Restoril	Transdermally	PO	IV
8.	NicoDerm CQ	Transdermally	PO	IV
9.	propofol	Transdermally	PO	IV
10.	Cymbalta	Transdermally	PO	IV

STUDENT NAME _____

DATE _____ INSTRUCTOR'S NAME _____

Identify whether the following are available parenterally, orally, or both (circle one).

1. haloperidol	Parenteral	Oral	Both
2. memantine	Parenteral	Oral	Both
3. Lunesta	Parenteral	Oral	Both
4. fluphenazine	Parenteral	Oral	Both
5. nortriptyline	Parenteral	Oral	Both
6. diazepam	Parenteral	Oral	Both
7. Serzone	Parenteral	Oral	Both
8. Thorazine	Parenteral	Oral	Both
9. Fiorinal	Parenteral	Oral	Both
10. Ativan	Parenteral	Oral	Both

Select the appropriate main use/drug class (circle one).

1. Concerta	Insomnia	ADHD	Seizure disorders
2. phenytoin	Insomnia	ADHD	Seizure disorders
3. valproic acid	Insomnia	ADHD	Seizure disorders
4. zaleplon	Insomnia	ADHD	Seizure disorders
5. Focalin XR	Insomnia	ADHD	Seizure disorders
6. temazepam	Insomnia	ADHD	Seizure disorders
7. gabapentin	Insomnia	ADHD	Seizure disorders
8. Tegretol	Insomnia	ADHD	Seizure disorders
9. zolpidem	Insomnia	ADHD	Seizure disorders

Select the appropriate main use/drug class (circle one).

		Alzheimer's	Parkinson's	Anxiety disorders
1.	benztropine	Alzheimer's	Parkinson's	Anxiety disorders
2.	galantamine	Alzheimer's	Parkinson's	Anxiety disorders
3.	Namenda	Alzheimer's	Parkinson's	Anxiety disorders
4.	BuSpar	Alzheimer's	Parkinson's	Anxiety disorders
5.	Carbidopa/levodopa	Alzheimer's	Parkinson's	Anxiety disorders
6.	clonazepam	Alzheimer's	Parkinson's	Anxiety disorders
7.	Mirapex	Alzheimer's	Parkinson's	Anxiety disorders
8.	meprobamate	Alzheimer's	Parkinson's	Anxiety disorders
9.	Librium	Alzheimer's	Parkinson's	Anxiety disorders
10.	rivastigmine	Alzheimer's	Parkinson's	Anxiety disorders

Identify whether the following questions are true or false (circle one).

1. Desflurane is a medication used for anesthesia.

   TRUE   FALSE

2. Relpax is given intravenously.

   TRUE   FALSE

3. Campral is used to help treat addictions.

   TRUE   FALSE

4. Lithium is used to treat seizure disorders.

   TRUE   FALSE

5. Mellaril is a brand name for thioridazine.

   TRUE   FALSE

6. Thiothixene is generic for Navane.

   TRUE   FALSE

7. Phenelzine is a medication used to treat anxiety disorders.

   TRUE   FALSE

8. Luvox is a brand name for fluvoxamine.

   TRUE   FALSE

9. Effexor is used to treat seizure disorders.

   TRUE   FALSE

10. Isocarboxazid is generic for Marplan.

    TRUE   FALSE

STUDENT NAME _____

DATE _____   INSTRUCTOR'S NAME _____

Select a common strength for the following medications.

1. acamprosate
   a. 30mg
   b. 300mg
   c. 333mg
   d. 350mg

2. Chantix
   a. 1000mg
   b. 100mg
   c. 10mg
   d. 1mg

3. Depakote
   a. 175mg
   b. 200mg
   c. 225mg
   d. 250mg

4. Focalin XR
   a. 10mg
   b. 25mg
   c. 50mg
   d. 100mg

5. Namenda
   a. 5mg
   b. 15mg
   c. 25mg
   d. 50mg

6. Ambien CR
   a. 12.5mg
   b. 25mg
   c. 50mg
   d. 100mg

7. carbidopa and levodopa
   a. 25mg/250mg
   b. 50mg/500mg
   c. 100mg/500mg
   d. 65mg/650mg

8. Mirapex
   a. 0.25mg
   b. 2.5mg
   c. 25mg
   d. 250mg

9. BuSpar
   a. 10mg
   b. 100mg
   c. 1000mg
   d. 2000mg

10. Provigil
    a. 10mg
    b. 50mg
    c. 75mg
    d. 100mg

11. Relpax
    a. 5mg
    b. 10mg
    c. 25mg
    d. 40mg

12. Strattera
    a. 5mg
    b. 18mg
    c. 50mg
    d. 180mg

13. Razadyne
    a. 1mg
    b. 2mg
    c. 4mg
    d. 10mg

14. Effexor XR
    a. 10mg
    b. 75mg
    c. 200mg
    d. 500mg

15. mirtazapine
    a. 30mg
    b. 40mg
    c. 50mg
    d. 60mg

8. EXERCISES

DISCUSSION AND CRITICAL THINKING QUESTIONS

1. Why are some ADHD medications only given 5 days per week and only during the school year?

2. Which categories of nervous system medications would make sense to be dosed PRN, and which would make sense to take regularly?

3. How do migraine headaches differ from stress or sinus headaches?

4. Which nervous system conditions are likely to respond to lifestyle changes?

STUDENT NAME _____

DATE _____   INSTRUCTOR'S NAME _____

5. Why might someone need more than one kind of nervous system medication to treat only one condition?

_____

_____

_____

_____

SAMPLE PRESCRIPTIONS

DEA # BD0000000

John Doe, M.D.
123 Any Street
Any Town, Any State 00000
Tel. (123) 456-7890   Fax. (123) 456-1234

NAME _Stephen Jackson_____

ADDRESS _573 Derby Ln._____

Rx   Focalin XR 5 mg   #30

Sig: T I T PO QAM

_____   J. Doe   M.D.
                                (Signature)

REFILL _NR_____

1. What is the generic name for Focalin XR?

_____

_____

_____

2. How would you translate the Sig code into plain English so that the patient could understand the directions for use?

_____

_____

_____

_____

_____

3. How many refills are given on this prescription?

_____

_____

_____

_____

_____

4. Is this a controlled substance, and if so, what is its DEA schedule?

_____

_____

_____

_____

_____

_____

5. What common condition(s) does this medication treat?

_____

_____

_____

_____

_____

Technician Tip

Most medications used to treat ADHD are listed as C-II substances and therefore will likely have additional record-keeping requirements and refill restrictions in your state. Atomoxetine is one exception; it is used to treat ADHD but is not a controlled substance. ℞

STUDENT NAME _____

DATE _____ INSTRUCTOR'S NAME _____

DEA # BD0000000

John Doe, M.D.
123 Any Street
Any Town, Any State 00000
Tel. (123) 456-7890   Fax. (123) 456-1234

NAME *Teddy Frederick*

ADDRESS *138 S. Front St.*

Rx *Suboxone 8-2mg #30 (thirty)*

Sig: *T 1 T PO QD*
XD0000000

_____ M.D.
J. Doe
(Signature)

REFILL *NR*

---

1. What is the generic name for Suboxone?

   _____

   _____

2. How would you translate the Sig code into plain English so that the patient could understand the directions for use?

   _____

   _____

   _____

3. How many refills are given on this prescription?

_____

_____

_____

_____

4. What other common strengths are available for Suboxone?

_____

_____

_____

_____

5. What is a common use for this medication?

_____

_____

_____

_____

Technician Tip

Physicians must write their "X" DEA number on a prescription for Suboxone for it to be filled. The "X" DEA number is different from a physician's DEA number; the "X" DEA number will start with an "X." It is acceptable to fill the prescription without the "X" DEA number if the prescription clearly indicates that the medication is to be used for pain, and not to help treat an addiction. If there is any confusion as to whether it is appropriate to fill a prescription for Suboxone, check with your pharmacist. ℞

STUDENT NAME _____

DATE _____ INSTRUCTOR'S NAME _____

DEA # BD0000000

John Doe, M.D.
123 Any Street
Any Town, Any State 00000
Tel. (123) 456-7890   Fax. (123) 456-1234

NAME *Phil Toothman* _____

ADDRESS *1421 Park Circle* _____

℞ *Zyprexa 10mg #30*

Sig: *T 1 T PO QD*

_____ *J. Doe*   M.D.
                    (Signature)

REFILL *RFx3*

NDC 0002-4117-30
30 Tablets   No. 4117
ZyPREXA
*Olanzapine
Tablets*   LILLY
                4117
10 mg   **Rx only**
Medication Guide is to be
dispensed to patients.
zyprexa.com   *Lilly*

1. What is the generic name for Zyprexa?

   _____

   _____

2. How would you translate the Sig code into plain English so that the patient could understand the directions for use?

   _____

   _____

   _____

3. How many refills are given on this prescription?

4. What other common strengths are available for Zyprexa?

5. What is a common use for this medication?

Respiratory Medications

9

KEY TERMS

Allergy

Asthma

Bronchodilator

Bronchospasm

Chronic obstructive pulmonary disease (COPD)

Expectorate

Inhalation

Inhaler

Metered-dose inhaler (MDI)

Nebulizer

Wheeze

LEARNING OBJECTIVES

After completing this chapter, the student will be able to:

1. Describe the basic anatomy and physiology of the respiratory system
2. Explain the therapeutic effect of common respiratory medications
3. List the brand and generic names for common respiratory medications
4. List uses of common respiratory medications
5. Identify available dosage forms for common respiratory medications
6. Identify routes of administration for common respiratory medications
7. Identify usual doses for common respiratory medications
8. List common side effects of frequently prescribed respiratory medications
9. List abbreviations for terms associated with the use of medication therapy for common diseases affecting the respiratory system
10. Describe alternative therapies commonly used to treat diseases of the respiratory system

Basic Anatomy and Physiology of the Respiratory System

The respiratory system works to provide oxygen to the body through the lungs and also to expel carbon dioxide. The organs of the respiratory system are shown in Figure 9-1.

Structurally, the respiratory system has two parts: 1) the upper respiratory tract; and 2) the lower respiratory tract. The upper respiratory tract includes the nasal cavity, choana, nostril, hard palate, soft palate, nasopharynx, oropharynx, epiglottis, laryngopharynx, larynx, and esophagus. The lower respiratory tract includes the trachea, carina of trachea, upper lung lobes, primary bronchi, secondary bronchi, tertiary bronchi, as well as horizontal fissures, oblique fissures, pleural cavity, visceral pleura, parietal pleura, and the diaphragm.

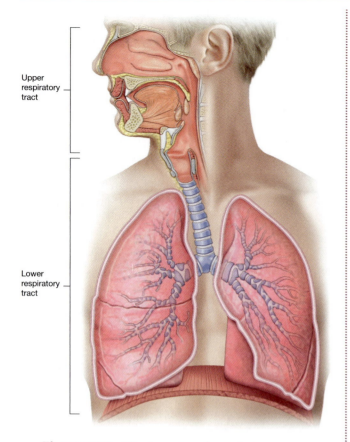

Upper respiratory tract

Lower respiratory tract

Figure 9-1. The lungs and respiratory tract.

Air enters the upper respiratory tract and progresses to the lower respiratory tract through the trachea. The trachea branch into two primary bronchi, and each primary bronchus branches into secondary bronchi. The secondary bronchi continue to branch into tertiary bronchi, quaternary bronchi, and more, until the branches become bronchioles, which are passageways less than 1 mm in diameter. Terminal bronchioles lead to respiratory bronchioles that contain alveoli in their walls. Oxygen diffuses from the respiratory system to the circulatory system when it passes from alveoli into pulmonary capillary beds. Also, carbon dioxide, a waste product, is passed from the circulatory system to the alveoli so it can be exhaled using the same passageways. Figure 9-2 shows the proximity of pulmonary capillary beds to alveoli that are embedded in the walls of respiratory bronchioles.

Knowing the following terms will be helpful as you learn about the medications used to treat conditions affecting the respiratory tract.

Allergy: A physical response to a substance, situation, or physical state that is exaggerated compared with what the average person experiences

Asthma: A chronic lung disorder characterized by episodes of obstructed breathing

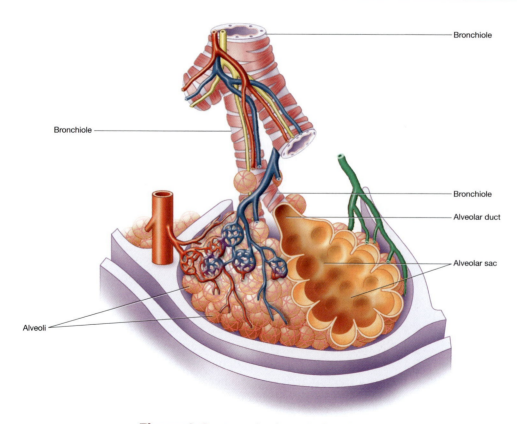

Bronchiole

Bronchiole

Bronchiole

Alveolar duct

Alveolar sac

Alveoli

Figure 9-2. Bronchiole and alveolar sac.

Bronchodilator: A device or medication that expands or dilates the airways

Bronchospasm: A muscle contraction of the airway muscles that constricts breathing

Chronic Obstructive Pulmonary Disease (COPD): A form of lung disease characterized by airway narrowing or obstruction and a slower rate of breathing

Expectorate: To spit out

Inhalation: The process by which air or medication is taken into the lungs

Inhaler: A device used to deliver medication to the lungs via inhalation

Metered-Dose Inhaler (MDI): An often pocket-sized device that delivers a fixed dose of medication upon each use

Nebulizer: A device that converts a liquid solution into a fine mist to deliver medication to the lungs via inhalation

Wheeze: To breathe with difficulty, often accompanied by a whistling sound

Primer on Pharmacologic Actions of Respiratory Medications

Respiratory medications are used to treat a wide variety of conditions associated with the respiratory tract. Respiratory medications are used to treat asthma and chronic obstructive pulmonary disease (COPD), as well as coughs and colds, allergies, and other conditions associated with the respiratory system.

Many of the medications used to treat asthma and COPD are administered through inhalers. Inhalers are devices that allow the drugs to be delivered directly to the site of action, generally through oral or nasal use. In the case of respiratory medications, inhalers generally target the lungs.

It is important for the pharmacy technician to know that not all inhalers have the same purpose. Some inhalers are called "rescue inhalers" and contain bronchodilators that are intended to open the breathing passages rapidly and to treat acute respiratory

distress. Other inhalers are used as maintenance medications that are intended to prevent breathing difficulties from occurring. Sometimes, oral anti-inflammatory steroids are needed to reduce inflammation of the breathing passages.

Coughs, colds, and allergies are treated with agents that are intended to provide the patient with relief from their symptoms. However, these agents do not cure the underlying condition that causes the symptoms.

℞ Cough suppressants are commonly used to treat most coughs

℞ Antihistamines have drying effects and are commonly used to treat allergies as well as runny noses associated with some colds; antihistamines are also used to treat itching conditions associated with allergic reactions

℞ Decongestants work to open upper respiratory breathing passages and are used to treat congestion that often accompanies colds and allergies

℞ Expectorants are used in combination with drinking water and work to thin mucus associated with coughs and colds, as well as other mucus-producing conditions, allowing the mucus to be coughed or spit out

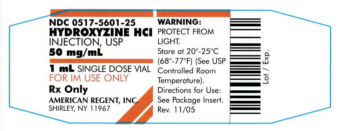

What is a common use for hydroxyzine?

Some common respiratory agents and their uses are listed in Table 9-1.

Table 9-1. Common Respiratory Agents and Their Uses

Generic Name	Brand Name	Dosage Form	Route	Common Use	Common Frequency	Common Strengths
beclomethasone	Beconase	Nasal spray	IN	Allergies, anti-inflammatory	b.i.d.	168mcg
ciclesonide	Omnaris	Nasal spray	IN	Allergies, anti-inflammatory	q.d.	50mg
cromolyn (OTC)	NasalCrom	Nasal spray	IN	Allergies	t.i.d.–q.i.d.	40mg
fluticasone	Veramyst, Flonase	Nasal spray	IN	Allergies, anti-inflammatory	q.d.	27.5mcg, 50mcg
levocetirizine	Xyzal	Tablet	PO	Allergies, antihistamine	q.d.	5mg
loratadine (OTC)	Claritin, Alavert	Tablet	PO	Allergies, antihistamine	q.d.	10mg
loratadine/ pseudoephedrine (OTC)	Claritin-D	Tablet	PO	Allergies, antihistamine + decongestant	q.d.	10mg/240mg
methylprednisolone	Medrol	Tablet	PO	Allergies, anti-inflammatory	q.d.–q.i.d.	4mg
mometasone	Nasonex	Nasal spray	IN	Allergies, anti-inflammatory	q.d.	100mcg
triamcinolone	Nasacort	Nasal spray	IN	Allergies, anti-inflammatory	q.d.	110mcg
budesonide	Rhinocort	Nasal spray	IN	Allergies anti-inflammatory	q.d.–b.i.d.	32mcg
cetirizine (OTC)	Zyrtec	Tablet	PO	Allergies antihistamine	q.d.	10mg
cetirizine/ pseudoephedrine (OTC)	Zyrtec-D	Tablet	PO	Allergies antihistamine + decongestant	b.i.d.	5/120mg
chlorpheniramine (OTC)	Chlor-Trimeton	Tablet	PO	Allergies, antihistamine	q.4–6h	4mg
desloratadine (OTC)	Clarinex	Tablet	PO	Allergies, antihistamine	q.d.	5mg
diphenhydramine (OTC)	Benadryl	Capsul/tablet/ liquid/ parenteral	PO/IV	Allergies, antihistamine	q.4–6h	25mg
fexofenadine	Allegra	Tablet	PO	Allergies, antihistamine	q.d.–b.i.d.	60mg, 180mg
fexofenadine/ pseudoephedrine	Allegra-D	Tablet	PO	Allergies, Antihistamine + decongestant	q.d.–b.i.d.	60/120mg, 60/240mg
hydroxyzine	Vistaril	Capsule	PO	Allergies, antihistamine	t.i.d.–q.i.d.	25mg
promethazine	Phenergan	Tablet, liquid	PO	Allergies, antihistamine	q.d.–t.i.d.	12.5mg, 25mg, 6.25mg/5ml

(Continued)

Table 9-1. Common Respiratory Agents and Their Uses (Continued)

Generic Name	Brand Name	Dosage Form	Route	Common Use	Common Frequency	Common Strengths
azelastine	Astelin	Nasal spray	IN	Allergies, antihistamine	b.i.d.	137mcg
epinephrine	EpiPen	Parenteral	IM/SQ	Anaphylaxis, bronchodilator	PRN	0.15mg, 0.3mg
montelukast	Singulair	Tablet	PO	Asthma,	q.d.	4mg, 10mg
zafirlukast	Accolate	Tablet	PO	Asthma,	b.i.d.	10mg, 20mg
zileuton	Zyflo-CR	Tablet	PO	Asthma	b.i.d.	600mg
beclomethasone	QVAR	Inhaler	PO	Asthma, anti-inflammatory	b.i.d.	40mcg, 80mcg
budesonide	Pulmicort MDI	Inhaler	PO	Asthma, anti-inflammatory	q.d.–b.i.d.	200mcg
budesonide (nebulizer)	Pulmicort Respules	Solution	PO	Asthma, anti-inflammatory	q.d.–b.i.d.	0.25mg, 0.5mg, 1mg
ciclesonide	Alvesco	Inhaler	PO	Asthma, Anti-inflammatory	b.i.d.	80mcg, 160mcg
flunisolide	AeroBid	Inhaler	PO	Asthma, anti-inflammatory	b.i.d.	250mcg
fluticasone	Flovent HFA	Inhaler	PO	Asthma, anti-inflammatory	b.i.d.	44mcg, 110mcg, 220mcg
fluticasone/ salmeterol	Advair Diskus	Inhaler	PO	Asthma, anti-inflammatory	b.i.d.	100/50, 250/50, 500/50
mometasone furoate	Asmanex	Inhaler	PO	Asthma, anti-inflammatory	q.d.–b.i.d.	220mcg
prednisolone	Orapred	Liquid	PO	Asthma, anti-inflammatory	q.d.–b.i.d.	15mg/5ml
theophylline	Theo-24	Capsule	PO	Asthma, bronchodilator	q.d.	100mg, 200mg, 300mg, 400mg
theophylline	Theophylline	Parenteral	IV	Asthma, bronchodilator	Continuous	200mg, 400mg, 800mg
albuterol	ProAir HFA	Inhaler	PO	Asthma, bronchodilator	PRN	90mcg
albuterol	Proventil HFA	Inhaler	PO	Asthma, bronchodilator	PRN	90mcg
albuterol	Ventolin HFA	Inhaler	PO	Asthma, COPD bronchodilator	PRN	90mcg

(Continued)

Table 9-1. Common Respiratory Agents and Their Uses (Continued)

Generic Name	Brand Name	Dosage Form	Route	Common Use	Common Frequency	Common Strengths
albuterol (nebulizer)	AccuNeb	Solution	PO	Asthma, COPD bronchodilator	PRN	0.63 mg, 1.25mg
budesonide/formoterol	Symbicort	Inhaler	PO	Asthma, COPD Anti-inflammatory	b.i.d.	80/4.5mcg, 160/4.5mcg
formoterol	Foradil	Inhaler	PO	Asthma, COPD bronchodilator	b.i.d.	12mcg
levalbuterol	Xopenex HFA	Inhaler	PO	Asthma, COPD bronchodilator	PRN	45mcg
levalbuterol (nebulizer)	Xopenex	Solution	PO	Asthma, COPD bronchodilator	PRN	0.31mg, 0.63mg, 1.25mg
salmeterol	Serevent	Inhaler	PO	Asthma, COPD bronchodilator	b.i.d.	50mcg
tiotropium	Spiriva	Inhaler	PO	COPD, bronchodilator	q.d.	18mcg
ipratropium	Atrovent	Inhaler	PO	COPD, bronchodilator	q.i.d.	18mcg
ipratropium/albuterol	Combivent	Inhaler	PO	COPD, bronchodilator	q.i.d.	103/18mcg
guaifenesin/codeine	Robitussin AC, Cheratussin AC	Liquid	PO	Cough expectorant + antitussive (C-V)	q.4h	100mg/10mg
guaifenesin/pseudoephedrine (OTC)	Mucinex-D	Tablet	PO	Cough expectorant + decongestant	b.i.d.–q.i.d.	600/60mg
promethazine/codeine	Phenergan with Codeine	Liquid	PO	Cough Antihistamine + antitussive (C-V)	q.4–6h	6.25mg/10mg
promethazine/dextromethorphan	Promethazine DM	Liquid	PO	Cough Antihistamine + antitussive	q.4–6h	6.25mg/15mg
camphor, eucalyptus, menthol (OTC)	Vicks VapoRub	Ointment	Topical	Cough suppressant, pain relief	Use up to t.i.d. PRN	4.8%, 1.2%, 2.6%
guaifenesin (OTC)	Mucinex	Tablet	PO	Cough, expectorant	q.12h	600mg, 1200mg
guaifenesin (OTC)	Robitussin	Liquid	PO	Cough, Expectorant	q.4h	200mg, 400mg
guaifenesin/dextromethorphan (OTC)	Robitussin DM	Liquid	PO	Cough, expectorant + antitussive	q.4h	100mg/10mg
phenylephrine/chlorpheniramine/dextromethorphan	C-Phen DM	Liquid	PO	Cough, decongestant + antihistamine + antitussive	q.4–6h	12.5/4/15mg

(Continued)

Table 9-1. Common Respiratory Agents and Their Uses *(Continued)*

Generic Name	Brand Name	Dosage Form	Route	Common Use	Common Frequency	Common Strengths
benzonatate	Tessalon	Capsule	PO	Cough, antitussive	t.i.d.–Q4H	100mg, 200mg
chlorpheniramine/ hydrocodone (CIII)	Tussionex	Liquid	PO	Cough, allergy antihistamine + antitussive	Q12H	10mg/8mg/5ml
oxymetazoline (OTC)	Afrin	Nasal spray	IN	Decongestant	b.i.d.	0.05%
phenylephrine (OTC)	Sudafed-PE	Tablet	PO	Decongestant	q.4–6h	10mg
pseudoephedrine (BTC)	Sudafed	Tablet	PO	Decongestant	q.4–6h	30mg
acetaminophen, chlorpheniramine, dextromethorphan, phenylephrine (OTC)	Theraflu Nighttime Severe Cough and Cold	Caplet	PO	Multisymptom cold relief	q.4h	325mg/2mg/10mg/5mg
acetaminophen, dextromethorphan, and phenylephrine (OTC)	Theraflu Daytime Severe Cold and Cough	Caplet	PO	Multisymptom cold relief	q.4h	325mg/10mg/5mg
acetaminophen, dextromethorphan, and phenylephrine (OTC)	DayQuil Cold and Flu	Liquid	PO	Multisymptom cold relief	q.4h	325mg/10mg/5mg
acetaminophen, dextromethorphan, doxylamine (OTC)	NyQuil	Liquid	PO	Multisymptom cold relief	q.6h	325mg/15mg/6.25mg

Technician Tip

Behind-the-counter (BTC) medications, such as pseudoephedrine, are considered a special class of over-the-counter (OTC) medications that are stored behind the pharmacy counter. Drugs classified as BTC have additional record-keeping requirements in many states. Additionally, patients may need to provide a photo ID and other information based on the laws in your state. If you are unsure of the BTC requirements in your state, check with your pharmacist. ℞

Dosage Forms, Routes of Administration, and Usual Doses for Common Respiratory Medications

Although tablets and capsules are used to treat many conditions, some respiratory conditions are treated with liquid medications, IV medications, and inhaled medications. For instance, theophylline can be given as a tablet, capsule, or liquid on an ongoing basis to prevent asthma attacks. Additionally, if a patient is in the hospital and not able to take medication by mouth, theophylline can also be given in IV form for the same use.

To get medication quickly and directly to the lungs, a solution of medication may be placed in a machine called a nebulizer. The nebulizer turns the liquid medication into a vapor that can be breathed in by the patient to deliver the medication directly to the lungs. The same concept is seen more commonly with inhalers, which are pocket-sized devices that emit a vapor of medicine for the patient to breathe. Patients often take 1 or 2 inhalations or "puffs" at a time, sometimes several times a day. Inhalers can be used on a regular basis to prevent breathing difficulties, or in a more emergent setting when a person is not breathing properly.

Many times, there is an underlying condition, such as a bad cough or allergy, that is preventing a patient from breathing properly, and treatment of that underlying condition can also help. In this regard, nasal sprays can sometimes be used to help air pass more easily through the nose if congestion is an issue.

Common Side Effects of Respiratory Medications

Inhalers, particularly the short-acting or "rescue" inhalers, may cause a patient to become excited or have a fast heartbeat. Medications used to treat allergies may cause drowsiness, particularly diphenhydramine (Benadryl), which can cause so much drowsiness that it is sometimes used to help people sleep. Cough syrups may contain alcohol and controlled substances, which may cause drowsiness. It is therefore recommended that patients not consume alcohol with cough syrups.

Technician Tip

It is important to label the inhaler box as well as the inhaler itself, if possible. Check with your pharmacist to see how he or she would like you to label inhalers, and be careful that your label does not cover up any important information on the packaging or interfere with the operation of the inhaler. Your pharmacist may have differing preferences for oral inhalers compared with nasal inhalers. ℞

Technician Tip

Some cough syrups contain controlled substances, such as codeine. Controlled substances have limits on refills and may have other dispensing and record-keeping requirements in your state. Products containing hydrocodone are often Schedule III, whereas products containing codeine are often Schedule V. ℞

Terminology and Common Abbreviations Used with Common Respiratory Medications

See Table 2-1, page 13, for abbreviations.

What's in a name?

Table 9-2. Examples of USAN Stems for Respiratory Medications		
Stem	**Description**	**Example**
-ast	Antiasthmatics/antiallergics (leukotriene biosynthesis inhibitors)	zafirlukast
-(a)tadine	Tricyclic histaminic-H1 receptor antagonists, loratadine derivatives	desloratadine
-astine	Antihistaminics (histamine H1 receptor antagonists)	azelastine
-terol	Bronchodilators (phenethylamine derivatives)	albuterol

Sample Prescription for Respiratory Medications

DEA # BD0000000

John Doe, M.D.
123 Any Street
Any Town, Any State 00000
Tel. (123) 456-7890   Fax. (123) 456-1234

NAME ___ Eva Williams ___

ADDRESS ___ 938 Dayton Ave. ___

℞ ___ Albuterol HFA # 1 MDI ___

Sig: ___ Inhale 1-2 puffs Q4-6H PRN ___

___ J. Doe ___ M.D.
(Signature)

REFILL ___ NR ___

The above prescription should be interpreted as: One albuterol metered-dose inhaler. Inhale 1 or 2 puffs every 4 to 6 hours as needed, with no refills. Brand names for albuterol MDI are ProAir HFA, Proventil HFA, and Ventolin HFA.

Technician Tip

Some respiratory medications will have ranges on the prescription. For instance, 1–2 puffs, or 4–6 hours, as shown on this prescription. Patients may ask about the ranges, and it is important for the patient to talk with the pharmacist to determine the most appropriate dosing. ℞

Technician Tip

To calculate the days supply for the medication, it is important to know how many inhalations of medication the metered dose inhaler provides. For example, Proventil HFA comes in an 18g container and provides 200 metered inhalations. Proventil HFA also comes with a dose counter so that patients can easily discern how many doses remain. ℞

Technician Tip

Albuterol is a common medication in a metered dose inhaler, but it can also be given using a nebulizer. If you are unsure as to whether the prescriber intended for the prescription to be for an inhaler, ask the pharmacist. ℞

Additional Therapies for Respiratory Conditions

Some respiratory issues may have preventable or treatable causes. For instance, if a patient has asthma that is worsened by allergies, distancing the patient from the source of the allergies can help. Keeping the house very clean and free of dust if there is a dust allergy or keeping the patient away from dogs or cats if there is a pet allergy may help to reduce allergy symptoms. Zicam produces several products containing zinc and/or other ingredients. These ingredients have been proposed to help treat common colds and may be effective in helping to treat or prevent a common cold.

Chapter Summary !

The purpose of the respiratory system is to deliver oxygen to the body and expel carbon dioxide. Many medications exist to help the body handle conditions associated with the respiratory tract, such as asthma, COPD, allergies, and even common coughs and colds.

℞ Inhalers are used to deliver medication, such as albuterol, directly to the lungs. These medications are often used to keep the lungs and airways open to treat asthma and COPD

℞ Antihistamines, such as loratadine and diphenhydramine, are used to treat the itching and sneezing effects of allergies. In some cases, they may also be used to treat a runny nose. Nasal sprays are also available to treat nasal symptoms of allergies

℞ Decongestants, such as pseudoephedrine and phenylephrine, are used to open up breathing passages. Some patients may self-treat their common colds with OTC decongestants

℞ Expectorants, such as guaifenesin, help to thin mucus, and antitussives, such as dextromethorphan, help to reduce the amount of coughing a person may experience

Products containing several medications (combination products) may be used when a person has several symptoms associated with his or her respiratory condition.

STUDENT NAME _____

DATE _____ INSTRUCTOR'S NAME _____

ANATOMY, PHYSIOLOGY, AND PHARMACOLOGY QUESTIONS

Identify whether the following are located in the upper or lower respiratory tract (circle one).

1.	Bronchi	Lower respiratory tract	Upper respiratory tract
2.	Nostril	Lower respiratory tract	Upper respiratory tract
3.	Esophagus	Lower respiratory tract	Upper respiratory tract
4.	Pleural cavity	Lower respiratory tract	Upper respiratory tract
5.	Diaphragm	Lower respiratory tract	Upper respiratory tract

Identify whether the following questions are true or false (circle one).

1. Alveoli exchange carbon dioxide for oxygen.

   TRUE FALSE

2. Inhalers are only used for instant rescue, not for prevention of symptoms.

   TRUE FALSE

3. Decongestants are used to treat common colds.

   TRUE FALSE

4. Expectorants help to reduce coughing.

   TRUE FALSE

5. Antihistamines treat stuffy noses.

   TRUE FALSE

MEDICATION QUESTIONS

Match the following brand-name products with their generic names.

1. _____ Ventolin HFA
2. _____ EpiPen
3. _____ Mucinex-D
4. _____ Xyzal
5. _____ Afrin
6. _____ Clarinex
7. _____ Orapred
8. _____ Vistaril

A. guaifenesin and dextromethorphan
B. hydroxyzine
C. epinephrine
D. levocetirizine
E. prednisone
F. oxymetazoline
G. albuterol
H. desloratadine

9. EXERCISES

9. _____ Serevent
10. _____ Spiriva
11. _____ Sudafed
12. _____ NyQuil
13. _____ Zyrtec-D
14. _____ Benadryl
15. _____ Vicks VapoRub
16. _____ QVAR

A. salmeterol
B. acetaminophen, dextromethorphan, and doxylamine
C. tiotropium
D. cetirizine and pseudoephedrine
E. beclomethasone
F. pseudoephedrine
G. diphenhydramine
H. camphor, eucalyptus, and menthol

17. _____ Rhinocort
18. _____ Beconase
19. _____ Medrol
20. _____ Asmanex
21. _____ Singulair
22. _____ Phenergan
23. _____ Alavert
24. _____ Zyflo-CR

A. methylprednisolone
B. montelukast
C. loratadine
D. beclomethasone
E. budesonide
F. promethazine
G. zileuton
H. mometasone

25. _____ Promethazine DM
26. _____ Phenergan with Codeine
27. _____ Theo-24
28. _____ Nasacort
29. _____ Accolate
30. _____ DayQuil Cold and Flu
31. _____ Theraflu Nighttime Severe Cough and Cold
32. _____ Astelin

A. triamcinolone
B. zafirlukast
C. promethazine and dextromethorphan
D. theophylline
E. azelastine
F. promethazine and codeine
G. acetaminophen, chlorpheniramine, dextromethorphan, and phenylephrine
H. acetaminophen, dextromethorphan, and phenylephrine

STUDENT NAME _____

DATE _____   INSTRUCTOR'S NAME _____

33. _____ Zyrtec

34. _____ Pulmicort

35. _____ NasalCrom

36. _____ Symbicort

37. _____ Tessalon

38. _____ Chlor-Trimeton

39. _____ Ventolin HFA

40. _____ Allegra

A.   benzonatate

B.   budesonide

C.   cromolyn

D.   albuterol

E.   budesonide and formoterol

F.   cetirizine

G.   fexofenadine

H.   chlorpheniramine

41. _____ Flovent HFA

42. _____ Mucinex

43. _____ Robitussin DM

44. _____ AeroBid

45. _____ Claritin-D

46. _____ Asmanex

47. _____ Xopenex

48. _____ Atrovent

A.   fluticasone

B.   guaifenesin and dextromethorphan

C.   loratadine and pseudoephedrine

D.   levalbuterol

E.   guaifenesin

F.   mometasone furoate

G.   flunisolide

H.   ipratropium

49. _____ Robitussin AC

50. _____ Combivent

51. _____ Advair Diskus

52. _____ Omnaris

53. _____ Tussionex

54. _____ Sudafed-PE

55. _____ C-Phen DM

56. _____ Symbicort

A.   ciclesonide

B.   budesonide and formoterol

C.   guaifenesin and codeine

D.   fluticasone and salmeterol

E.   ipratropium and albuterol

F.   chlorpheniramine and hydrocodone

G.   phenylephedrine, chlorpheniramine, and dextromethorphan

H.   phenylephrine

Select a common and appropriate frequency of administration (circle one).

1. Advair Diskus	q.d.	b.i.d.	q.4–6h	PRN
2. Nasacort	q.d.	b.i.d.	q.4–6h	PRN
3. AccuNeb	q.d.	b.i.d.	q.4–6h	PRN
4. promethazine DM	q.d.	b.i.d.	q.4–6h	PRN
5. Accolate	q.d.	b.i.d.	q.4–6h	PRN
6. Singulair	q.d.	b.i.d.	q.4–6h	PRN
7. Claritin	q.d.	b.i.d.	q.4–6h	PRN
8. Alvesco	q.d.	b.i.d.	q.4–6h	PRN
9. Symbicort	q.d.	b.i.d.	q.4–6h	PRN
10. Phenergan with codeine	q.d.	b.i.d.	q.4–6h	PRN
11. Xopenex	q.d.	b.i.d.	q.4–6h	PRN
12. Sudafed	q.d.	b.i.d.	q.4–6h	PRN
13. Serevent	q.d.	b.i.d.	q.4–6h	PRN
14. Zyflo-CR	q.d.	b.i.d.	q.4–6h	PRN
15. C-Phen DM	q.d.	b.i.d.	q.4–6h	PRN

Select the correct dosage form (circle one).

1. ProAir HFA	Nasal spray	Inhaler	Tablet	Liquid
2. Rhinocort	Nasal spray	Inhaler	Tablet	Liquid
3. Allegra	Nasal spray	Inhaler	Tablet	Liquid
4. AeroBid	Nasal spray	Inhaler	Tablet	Liquid
5. Robitussin DM	Nasal spray	Inhaler	Tablet	Liquid
6. Atrovent	Nasal spray	Inhaler	Tablet	Liquid
7. Foradil	Nasal spray	Inhaler	Tablet	Liquid
8. NyQuil	Nasal spray	Inhaler	Tablet	Liquid
9. Astelin	Nasal spray	Inhaler	Tablet	Liquid
10. Orapred	Nasal spray	Inhaler	Tablet	Liquid

STUDENT NAME _____

DATE _____ INSTRUCTOR'S NAME _____

Identify whether the following are available parenterally, orally, or both (circle one).

1.	Theophylline	Parenteral	Oral	Both
2.	Zyrtec	Parenteral	Oral	Both
3.	EpiPen	Parenteral	Oral	Both
4.	Benadryl	Parenteral	Oral	Both
5.	Tessalon	Parenteral	Oral	Both

Identify the level of control for the following medications (circle one).

1.	Robitussin DM	OTC	Rx	C-V
2.	Robitussin AC	OTC	Rx	C-V
3.	budesonide	OTC	Rx	C-V
4.	Clarinex	OTC	Rx	C-V
5.	Claritin	OTC	Rx	C-V
6.	diphenhydramine	OTC	Rx	C-V
7.	promethazine/codeine	OTC	Rx	C-V
8.	Singulair	OTC	Rx	C-V
9.	guaifenesin	OTC	Rx	C-V
10.	tiotropium	OTC	Rx	C-V

Select the appropriate main use/drug class (circle one).

1.	Sudafed-PE	Allergies	Asthma	Decongestant
2.	theophylline	Allergies	Asthma	Decongestant
3.	Xyzal	Allergies	Asthma	Decongestant
4.	Advair	Allergies	Asthma	Decongestant
5.	Ventolin HFA	Allergies	Asthma	Decongestant
6.	Afrin	Allergies	Asthma	Decongestant
7.	Clarinex	Allergies	Asthma	Decongestant
8.	Symbicort	Allergies	Asthma	Decongestant

9.	Rhinocort	Allergies	Asthma	Decongestant
10.	Singulair	Allergies	Asthma	Decongestant
11.	DayQuil Cold and Flu	COPD	Cough	Multisymptom cold relief
12.	Spiriva	COPD	Cough	Multisymptom cold relief
13.	Robitussin	COPD	Cough	Multisymptom cold relief
14.	NyQuil	COPD	Cough	Multisymptom cold relief
15.	Atrovent	COPD	Cough	Multisymptom cold relief
16.	Promethazine DM	COPD	Cough	Multisymptom cold relief
17.	Combivent	COPD	Cough	Multisymptom cold relief
18.	Tussionex	COPD	Cough	Multisymptom cold relief
19.	Theraflu Daytime Severe Cough and Cold	COPD	Cough	Multisymptom cold relief
20.	benzonatate	COPD	Cough	Multisymptom cold relief

Identify whether the following questions are true or false (circle one).

1. Albuterol and budesonide can be given using a nebulizer.
   TRUE   FALSE

2. Allegra-D is used to treat a cough.
   TRUE   FALSE

3. The generic name for Robitussin is guaifenesin.
   TRUE   FALSE

4. The generic name for Sudafed-PE is dextromethorphan.
   TRUE   FALSE

5. Theraflu Nighttime Severe Cough and Cold contains, among other medications, acetaminophen and dextromethorphan.
   TRUE   FALSE

6. Vicks VapoRub is applied topically.
   TRUE   FALSE

7. Robitussin DM contains, among other medications, codeine.
   TRUE   FALSE

8. Tessalon is a brand name for benzonatate.
   TRUE   FALSE

STUDENT NAME _____

DATE _____   INSTRUCTOR'S NAME _____

9. An EpiPen is used for the treatment of anaphylaxis.

TRUE   FALSE

10. Hydroxyzine is most frequently taken b.i.d.

TRUE   FALSE

Select a common strength for the following medications.

1. Asmanex

   a. 200mcg
   b. 220mcg
   c. 250mcg
   d. 280mcg

2. Xyzal

   a. 5mg
   b. 10mg
   c. 15mg
   d. 20mg

3. Spiriva

   a. 10mg
   b. 12mg
   c. 15mg
   d. 18mg

4. Ventolin HFA

   a. 80mcg
   b. 90mcg
   c. 100mcg
   d. 110mcg

5. salmeterol

   a. 10mcg
   b. 25mcg
   c. 50mcg
   d. 100mcg

6. chlorpheniramine

   a. 1mg
   b. 2mg
   c. 3mg
   d. 4mg

7. Pulmicort MDI

   a. 50mcg
   b. 100mcg
   c. 200mcg
   d. 500mcg

8. AccuNeb

   a. 0.75mg
   b. 1.0mg
   c. 1.25mg
   d. 1.5mg

9. methylprednisolone

   a. 1mg
   b. 4mg
   c. 8mg
   d. 16mg

10. Mucinex

   a. 600mg
   b. 800mg
   c. 1000mg
   d. 1200mg

11. phenylephrine

   a. 10mg
   b. 20mg
   c. 30mg
   d. 40mg

12. Atrovent

   a. 10mg
   b. 12mg
   c. 18mg
   d. 20mg

13. cromolyn

   a. 10mg
   b. 20mg
   c. 40mg
   d. 80mg

14. fexofenadine

   a. 60mg
   b. 75mg
   c. 100mg
   d. 150mg

15. montelukast

   a. 7mg
   b. 8mg
   c. 9mg
   d. 10mg

Select the best available answer for the following questions.

1. Zyrtec-D contains _____.

    a. cetirizine and pseudoephedrine
    b. guaifenesin and hydrocodone
    c. chlorpheniramine and hydrocodone
    d. loratadine and pseudoephedrine

2. Mucinex and Robitussin are both brand names for _____.

    a. chlorpheniramine
    b. cetirizine
    c. loratadine
    d. guaifenesin

3. Tessalon is commonly used to treat _____.

    a. allergies
    b. cough
    c. asthma
    d. COPD

4. Sudafed and Afrin are both drugs that are used as a(n) _____.

    a. bronchodilator
    b. cough suppressant
    c. decongestant
    d. antihistamine

5. What do Vistaril and Benadryl have in common? _____.

    a. Both are given IV
    b. Both are antihistamines
    c. Both are antitussives
    d. Both are taken only once daily

6. Robitussin DM and promethazine DM both contain, among other medications, _____.

    a. triamterene and hydrochlorothiazide
    b. moexipril and hydrochlorothiazide
    c. amlodipine and atorvastatin
    d. niacin and lovastatin

7. The generic name of Spiriva is _____.

    a. zileuton
    b. zafirlukast
    c. tiotropium
    d. triamcinolone

8. The proper route of administration of Afrin is _____, and its generic name is _____.

    a. IN, oxymetazoline
    b. IN, phenylephrine
    c. PO, oxymetazoline
    d. PO, phenylephrine

STUDENT NAME _____

DATE _____ INSTRUCTOR'S NAME _____

9. Sudafed is a brand name for _____, and Sudafed-PE is a brand name for _____.

    a. cetirizine, levocetirizine
    b. levocetirizine, cetirizine
    c. phenylephrine, pseudoephedrine
    d. pseudoephedrine, phenylephrine

10. C-Phen DM contains _____.

    a. phenylephrine and dextromethorphan
    b. phenylephrine, chlorpheniramine, and dextromethorphan
    c. chlorpheniramine and dextromethorphan
    d. guaifenesin and dextromethorphan

11. Diphenhydramine is generic for _____.

    a. Benadryl
    b. Clarinex
    c. Symbicort
    d. Advair

12. Tussionex is available as a _____.

    a. tablet
    b. liquid
    c. capsule
    d. spray

13. Fluticasone is a medication contained in which of the following brand-name products? _____

    a. Vicks VapoRub
    b. Veramyst
    c. Xopenex
    d. Asmanex

14. Proventil HFA, ProAir HFA, and Ventolin HFA each contain _____.

    a. albuterol
    b. budesonide
    c. beclomethasone
    d. cromolyn

15. Flonase is a brand name of _____.

    a. chlorpheniramine
    b. fluticasone
    c. triamcinolone
    d. azelastine

9. EXERCISES

DISCUSSION AND CRITICAL THINKING QUESTIONS

1. What are the dangers of a patient confusing a rescue inhaler with a maintenance inhaler?

2. What types of medications are used to control the symptoms of common colds? What are some examples of these medications?

3. What special record-keeping and storage requirements exist for products containing pseudoephedrine in your pharmacy?

4. In what ways might a person try to prevent allergies from becoming problematic?

5. If a patient uses a nebulizer at home, why might he or she also use an inhaler for the same medication?

STUDENT NAME _____

DATE _____ INSTRUCTOR'S NAME _____

SAMPLE PRESCRIPTIONS

DEA # BD0000000

John Doe, M.D.
123 Any Street
Any Town, Any State 00000
Tel. (123) 456-7890   Fax. (123) 456-1234

NAME _____ Sully Bakerson _____

ADDRESS _____ 1722 W. 14th Ave. _____

Rx   Spiriva #1 Inhaler

Sig: 1 puff QD

_____ J. Doe _____ M.D.
(Signature)

REFILL _____ NR _____

1. What is the generic name for Spiriva?

_____

_____

2. What is a common use for Spiriva?

_____

_____

3. How would you translate the Sig code into plain English so that the patient could understand the directions for use?

4. Spiriva, as carried by your pharmacy, comes with 30 capsules in a blister pack. Spiriva capsules are inserted into the inhaler device, punctured by the device, and the powder inside the capsule is inhaled. One capsule is used per inhalation. What is the days supply for this prescription?

Technician Tip

Spiriva is considered a dry powder inhaler. Blister packs of capsules come in the box with the inhaler that contains the medication. Capsules are placed into the inhaler, which are broken open by the inhaler, and the patient inhales the powder contained in the capsule. Spiriva capsules should not be swallowed. ℞

STUDENT NAME _____

DATE _____ INSTRUCTOR'S NAME _____

DEA # BD0000000

John Doe, M.D.
123 Any Street
Any Town, Any State 00000
Tel. (123) 456-7890   Fax. (123) 456-1234

NAME _____ Sam Melvin _____

ADDRESS _____ 1422 Sparrow Ln. _____

Rx   Robitussin AC #120ml

Sig: 1 tsp PO q4-6H PRN

_____ J. Doe _____ M.D.
(Signature)

REFILL _____ NR _____

---

1. What ingredients are included in Robitussin AC?

   _____

   _____

2. What is a common use for Robitussin AC?

   _____

   _____

Technician Tip

Some prescribers will use a combination of teaspoons and milliliters to describe the volume of the prescription. When calculating between the two forms of measurement, it is important to remember that 1 teaspoon is equivalent to 5 milliliters, and 1 ounce is equivalent to 30ml. The pharmacist may additionally discuss this conversion with the patient and show the patient exactly how to use a dosing spoon or dropper. **Rx**

3. How would you translate the Sig code into plain English so that the patient could understand the directions for use?

_____

_____

_____

_____

_____

4. What is the minimum days supply for this prescription?

_____

_____

_____

_____

5. How many ounces will you dispense to the patient?

_____

_____

_____

_____

_____

Technician Tip

Robitussin AC contains codeine, a controlled substance. your state may have additional record-keeping requirements, transfer limitations, and/or refill limitations for controlled substances. Check with your pharmacist if you are unsure of the legal issues surrounding controlled substances in your state. ℞

STUDENT NAME _____

DATE _____ INSTRUCTOR'S NAME _____

DEA # BD0000000

John Doe, M.D.
123 Any Street
Any Town, Any State 00000
Tel. (123) 456-7890   Fax. (123) 456-1234

NAME _____Stan McClark_____

ADDRESS ___1224 Colorado Blvd._____

Rx   Zyrtec-D #60

Sig: T 1 T PO BID

_____ J. Doe _____ M.D.
(Signature)

REFILL ___Rfx3___

---

1. What ingredients and strengths are included in Zyrtec-D?

   _____

   _____

2. What is a common use for Zyrtec-D?

   _____

   _____

   _____

3. How would you translate the Sig code into plain English so that the patient could understand the directions for use?

_____

_____

_____

_____

_____

4. What is the days supply for this prescription?

_____

_____

_____

_____

Technician Tip

Zyrtec-D is available both as a prescription and over the counter. Insurance companies will often cover Zyrtec-D if it is listed as a prescription, but not if it is bought over the counter. Additionally, because Zyrtec-D contains pseudoephedrine, it may be stored behind the counder and considered a behind-the-counter (BTC) medication. ℞

Gastrointestinal Medications

10

KEY TERMS

Alimentary canal

Digestion

Esophagus

Gallbladder

Gastrointestinal tract

Liver

Pancreas

Salivary glands

LEARNING OBJECTIVES

After completing this chapter, the student will be able to:

1. Describe the basic anatomy and physiology of the gastrointestinal system

2. Explain the therapeutic effects of common medications used to treat diseases of the gastrointestinal system

3. List the brand and generic names of common medications used to treat diseases of the gastrointestinal system

4. Identify available dosage forms for common gastrointestinal system medications

5. Identify routes of administration for common gastrointestinal system medications

6. Identify usual doses for common gastrointestinal system medications

7. List common side effects of frequently prescribed gastrointestinal system medications

8. Define medical terms commonly used when treating diseases of the gastrointestinal system

9. List abbreviations for terms associated with the use of medication therapy for common diseases affecting the gastrointestinal system

10. Describe alternative therapies commonly used to treat diseases of the gastrointestinal system

11. List products for the gastrointestinal system that are available over-the-counter and their strengths

Basic Anatomy and Physiology of the Gastrointestinal System

Digestion is the term for the body process of breaking down food into simpler chemicals. Food travels through the gastrointestinal (GI) tract as part of the process of digestion. The alimentary canal is another term for the GI tract. Accessory organs are also associated with the process of digestion and include the teeth and tongue, salivary glands, liver and gall-bladder, and pancreas. The digestive system consists of the GI tract along with the accessory organs. Figure 10-1 shows the organs of the digestive system.

Some parts of the digestive system shown include the oral cavity, tongue, gallbladder, duodenum, ascending colon of large intestine, esophagus, stomach, transverse colon, descending colon, small intestine, sigmoid colon, rectum, anal canal, and anus.

Knowing the following terms will be helpful as you learn about the medications used to treat conditions affecting the GI system.

Alimentary canal: another term for the gastrointestinal tract or organs through which food travels as part of digestion

Digestion: the process of breaking down food into simpler chemicals

Esophagus: passage for food to travel to the stomach

Gallbladder: accessory organ associated with the process of digestion

Gastrointestinal tract: the system of organs through which food travels during digestion

Liver: accessory organ associated with the process of digestion

Pancreas: accessory organ associated with the process of digestion

Salivary glands: accessory organ associated with the process of digestion

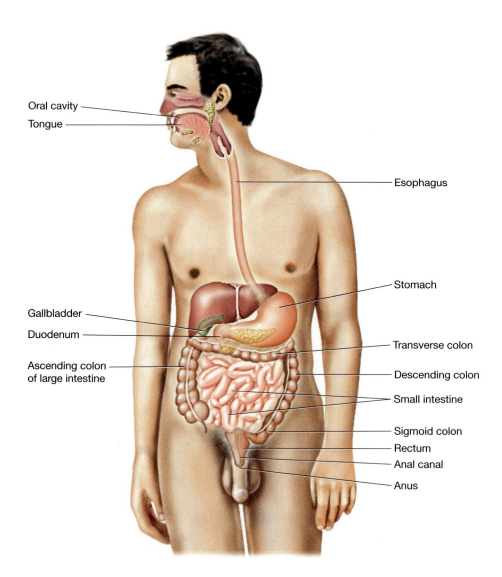

Oral cavity
Tongue
Esophagus
Stomach
Gallbladder
Duodenum
Transverse colon
Ascending colon of large intestine
Descending colon
Small intestine
Sigmoid colon
Rectum
Anal canal
Anus

Figure 10-1. Organs of the digestive system.

Primer on Pharmacologic Actions of Gastrointestinal Agents

Gastrointestinal agents are used to treat conditions of the GI tract. The most commonly treated conditions include constipation, diarrhea, gastroesophageal reflux, heartburn and indigestion, nausea and vomiting, obesity, spasms, ulcerative colitis, and ulcers. Additionally, some GI medications are used for cleansing the bowel before a gastrointestinal examination or surgery.

Constipation is a condition characterized by the infrequent passage of dry, hardened feces. Stimulant laxatives, such as bisacodyl (Dulcolax), are one type of medication used to treat constipation and produce their action by increasing movement in the bowels. Stimulant laxatives are often prescribed before rectal or bowel examinations or surgery. Osmotic laxatives such as polyethylene glycol 3350 (MiraLAX) can also be used to treat constipation and cause water to be retained with the stool to soften the stools so a bowel movement can be easier. Stool softeners, such as docusate (Colace), can also help with constipation by softening the stools without increasing stimulant effects.

Diarrhea is a condition of abnormally frequent bowel movements in which the stools may be accompanied by more liquid. Antidiarrheal medications such as loperamide (Imodium) work to decrease the frequency of bowel movements, as does Lomotil (diphenoxylate and atropine).

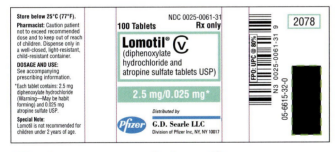

What is a common use for Lomotil?

Heartburn and indigestion can be symptoms of too much acid in the stomach. Antacids such as calcium carbonate (Tums) work directly in the stomach toneutralize acid.

If heartburn becomes more severe or frequent, a patient may have gastroesophageal reflux disease (GERD). Gastroesophageal reflux disease is a condition in which acid backs up from the stomach to cause heartburn as well as injury to the esophagus. Metoclopramide (Reglan) is an example of a drug that is used to speed the movement of food through the GI tract.

Obesity is a common condition in today's society and is associated with excessive accumulation and storage of fat in the body. Two types of medications are associated with treating obesity. Phentermine (Adipex-P) is an example of a drug that can help with obesity by reducing the appetite. Orlistat (Xenical) is a medication that blocks the absorption in the intestines of some of the fat in foods, so that there is a decrease in calories absorbed from food that has been eaten.

Gastrointestinal spasms can be symptomatic of some disorders of the GI tract. Hyoscyamine (Levsin) is an example of a drug used to control spasms in the GI tract by reducing GI motility as well as decreasing the production of stomach fluids. Hyoscyamine can also be used to treat spasmodic conditions associated with some other organs, such as the bladder.

Ulcerative colitis is a condition affecting the lining of the large intestine and is associated with inflammation and pain. Mesalamine (Asacol) is an example of a specialized anti-inflammatory medication used to decrease production of the substances associated with inflammation and pain in the intestine.

Peptic ulcers are more commonly known as ulcers and are characterized by damaged tissue in the wall of the stomach. The damage is sometimes caused by excess stomach acid production but can also be caused by an infection of *Helicobacter pylori* or by chronic use of nonsteroidal anti-inflammatory agents (NSAIDs). Drugs such as cimetidine (Tagamet) and lansoprazole (Prevacid) work in different ways to reduce the production of stomach acid. In the case of ulcers caused by *H. pylori* infections, drug combinations that include medications to reduce acid productions along with antibiotics are prescribed, such as lansoprazole with the antibiotics amoxicillin and clarithromycin (Prevpac). For some patients with NSAID-induced ulcers, the medication misoprostol (Cytotec) can be prescribed to decrease stomach acid production caused by the NSAID (see Chapter 7 for examples of NSAID medications).

Nausea and vomiting can be caused by many illnesses and also by chemotherapy and radiation therapy for cancer treatment and by surgery. Ondansetron (Zofran) is an example of a medication used to prevent nausea and vomiting caused by chemotherapy, radiation therapy, and surgery.

Ondansetron works by blocking the action of a natural substance that may be the cause the nausea and vomiting.

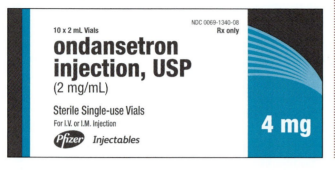

Some common gastrointestinal agents and their uses are listed in Table 10-1.

What is a common use for ondansetron?

Table 10-1. Common Gastrointestinal Agents and Their Uses

Generic Name	Brand Name	Dosage Form	Route	Common Use	Common Frequency	Common Strengths
polyethylene glycol electrolyte solution	CoLyte, GoLYTELY, TriLyte	Liquid	PO	Cleansing the bowel before a gastrointestinal examination or surgery	8oz q.10min until gone	2L, 4L
polyethylene glycol electrolyte solution and bisacodyl	HalfLytely and bisacodyl	Liquid	PO	Cleansing the bowel before a gastrointestinal examination or surgery	2 tablets as a single dose, 8oz q10min until gone	2L, 5mg
cimetidine (OTC)	Tagamet-HB	Tablet,	PO	Heartburn, indigestion, ulcers	b.i.d.–q.i.d.	200mg
famotidine (OTC)	Pepcid-AC	Tablet	PO	Heartburn, indigestion, ulcers	q.d.–b.i.d.	10mg
nizatidine (OTC)	Axid-AR	Tablet,	PO	Heartburn, indigestion, ulcers	q.d.–b.i.d.	75mg
ranitidine (OTC)	Zantac 75, Zantac 150	Tablet,	PO	Heartburn, indigestion, ulcers	q.d.–q.i.d.	75mg, 150mg,
cimetidine	Tagamet	Tablet, liquid	PO	Heartburn, indigestion, ulcers	b.i.d.–q.i.d.	200mg, 300mg, 400mg, 800mg, 300mg/5ml
famotidine	Pepcid	Tablet, parenteral	PO	Heartburn, indigestion, ulcers	q.d.–b.i.d.	10mg, 20mg, 40mg
nizatidine	Axid	Tablet, capsule, liquid	PO	Heartburn, indigestion, ulcers	q.d.–b.i.d.	75mg, 150mg, 300mg, 15mg/ml
ranitidine	Zantac	Tablet, liquid, parenteral	PO, IV, IM	Heartburn, indigestion, ulcers	q.d.–q.i.d.	75mg, 150mg, 300mg, 25mg/ml, 15mg/ml
bisacodyl (OTC)	Dulcolax	Tablet, suppository	PO, rectally	Laxative	5–15mg at once	5mg, 10mg

(Continued)

Table 10-1. Common Gastrointestinal Agents and Their Uses (Continued)

Generic Name	Brand Name	Dosage Form	Route	Common Use	Common Frequency	Common Strengths
polyethylene glycol 3350 (OTC)	MiraLAX	Powder for solution	PO	Osmotic laxative	17g in 4–8 oz beverage q.d.	17g
docusate (OTC)	Colace	Tablet, capsule, liquid, enema	PO, rectally	Stool softener	q.d.–q.i.d.	50mg, 100mg, 250mg, 20mg/5ml, 50mg/5ml, 283mg/5ml
lactulose	Chronulac, Duphalac, Enulose	Powder packet, solution	PO, rectally	Treating constipation	q.1–2h PRN	10g, 10g/15ml
lactulose	Kristalose	Liquid	PO	Treating constipation	20–30g q1–2h	10g/15ml
psyllium (OTC)	Metamucil	Capsule, powder	PO	Treating constipation	q.d.	500mg, 0.52g, 3.5g, 4.1g
diphenoxylate, atropine	Lomotil	Tablet, liquid	PO	Treating diarrhea (C-V)	PRN	2.5mg/0.025mg, 2.5mg/0.025mg/5ml
loperamide	Imodium	Caplet, capsule, liquid	PO	Treating diarrhea	PRN	2mg, 1mg/5ml
attapulgite	Kaopectate	Liquid	PO	Treating diarrhea	PRN	600mg/15ml, 750mg/15ml
Sandostatin	Octreotide	Parenteral	IV, IM, SQ	Treating diarrhea	b.i.d.–q.i.d., q.4weeks	0.05mg/ml, 0.2mg/ml, 20mg,
loperamide (OTC)	Imodium-AD	Caplet, capsule, liquid	PO	Treating diarrhea	PRN	2mg
loperamide and simethicone (OTC)	Imodium advanced, Imodium multi-symptom relief	Tablet, caplet	PO	Treating diarrhea, flatulence, and bloating	PRN	2mg/125mg
simethicone (OTC)	Gas X	Tablet, capsule, strip, softgel, suspension	PO	Treating flatu-lence/bloating	q.i.d. PRN	40mg, 80mg, 125mg, 166mg, 180mg, 40mg/0.6ml
metoclopramide	Reglan	Tablet, liquid, parenteral	PO, IV, IM	Treating gastro-esophageal reflux	q.i.d.	5mg, 10mg, 5mg/5ml, 5mg/ml
bismuth, metronidazole, tetracycline	Helidac	Tablet/capsule	PO	Treating *H. pylori* infections associ-ated with ulcers	q.i.d.	262.4mg/250mg/500mg
lansoprazole, amoxicillin, clarithromycin	Prevpac	Tablet/capsule	PO	Treating H. pylori infections associ-ated with ulcers	b.i.d.	30mg/1g/500mg

(Continued)

Table 10-1. Common Gastrointestinal Agents and Their Uses *(Continued)*

Generic Name	Brand Name	Dosage Form	Route	Common Use	Common Frequency	Common Strengths
aluminum hydroxide, magnesium hydroxide (OTC)	Maalox	Liquid	PO	Treating heartburn and indigestion	PRN	225mg/200mg/5ml
aluminum hydroxide, magnesium hydroxide, simethicone (OTC)	Mylanta	Liquid	PO	Treating heartburn and indigestion	PRN	200mg/200mg/ 20mg/5ml
calcium carbonate (OTC)	Tums	Tablet	PO	Treating heartburn and indigestion	PRN	500mg, 750mg, 1000mg
calcium carbonate, magnesium hydroxide (OTC)	Rolaids	Tablet	PO	Treating heartburn and indigestion	PRN	550mg/110mg
phenylephrine (OTC)	Preparation H	Cream, ointment, suppository	Rectally	Treating hemorrhoids	PRN up to q.i.d.	0.25%
meclizine (OTC)	Antivert, Bonine	Tablet, caplet	PO	Treating motion sickness, vertigo	q.d.–b.i.d.	12.5mg, 25mg
dolasetron	Anzemet	Tablet, parenteral	PO, IV	Treating nausea and vomiting	PRN	50mg, 100mg, 20mg/ml
granisetron	Kytril, Sancuso	Tablet, liquid, patch parenteral	PO, IV, topical	Treating nausea and vomiting	PRN	1mg, 3.1mg/24hr, 2mg/10ml, 1mg/ml
ondansetron	Zofran	Tablet, parenteral	PO, IV	Treating nausea and vomiting	PRN	4mg, 8mg, 24mg, 2mg/ml
prochlorperazine	Compazine	Tablet, suppository	PO, rectally	Treating nausea and vomiting	b.i.d.–q.i.d.	5mg, 10mg, 25mg
promethazine	Phenergan, Promethegan	Tablet, liquid, suppository, parenteral	PO, IV, IM, rectally	Treating nausea and vomiting	q.i.d.	12.5mg, 25mg 50mg, 6.25mg/5ml, 25mg/ml, 50mg/ml
misoprostol	Cytotec	Tablet	PO	Treating NSAID-induced ulcers	q.i.d.	100mcg, 200mcg
orlistat (OTC)	Alli, Xenical	Capsule	PO	Treating obesity	t.i.d.	60mg, 120mg
phentermine (CIV)	Adipex-P	Tablet, capsule	PO	Treating obesity	q.d., t.i.d.	15mg, 30mg, 37.5mg
dicyclomine	Bentyl	Tablet, capsule, liquid, parenteral	PO, IM	Treating spasms	q.i.d.	10mg, 20mg, 10mg/5ml, 10mg/ml
hyoscyamine	Anaspaz, Levbid, Levsin, NuLev	Tablet, liquid, parenteral	PO, IV, IM, SQ	Treating spasms	q.4h, q.i.d.	0.125mg, 0.375mg, 0.125mg/5ml, 0.5mg/ml
mesalamine	Asacol, Canasa, Lialda, Pentasa, Rowasa	Tablet, capsule, liquid, suppository	PO, rectally	Treating ulcerative colitis	q.d., t.i.d., q.i.d.	250mg, 375mg, 400mg, 500mg, 800mg, 1000mg, 1200mg, 4g/60ml

(Continued)

Table 10-1. Common Gastrointestinal Agents and Their Uses *(Continued)*

Generic Name	Brand Name	Dosage Form	Route	Common Use	Common Frequency	Common Strengths
sulfasalazine	Azulfidine	Tablet	PO	Treating ulcerative colitis	q.8h	500mg
sucralfate	Carafate	Tablet, liquid	PO	Treating ulcers	q.i.d.	1g, 1g/10ml
dexlansoprazole	Dexilant	Capsule	PO	Ulcers, gastrointestinal reflux	q.d.	30mg, 60mg
esomeprazole	Nexium	Capsule, parenteral	PO, IV	ulcers, gastrointestinal reflux	q.d.	20mg, 40mg
lansoprazole	Prevacid	Capsule, powder, parenteral	PO, IV	ulcers, gastrointestinal reflux	q.d.	15mg, 30mg
lansoprazole (OTC)	Prevacid-24HR	Capsule	PO	ulcers, gastrointestinal reflux	q.d.	15mg
omeprazole	Prilosec	Capsule	PO	ulcers, gastrointestinal reflux	q.d.	20mg, 40mg
omeprazole (OTC)	Prilosec OTC	Tablet	PO	ulcers, gastrointestinal reflux	q.d.	20mg
pantoprazole	Protonix	Tablet, parenteral	PO, IV	ulcers, gastrointestinal reflux	q.d.	20mg, 40mg
rabeprazole	AcipHex	Tablet	PO	ulcers, gastrointestinal reflux	q.d.	20mg

Dosage Forms, Routes of Administration, and Usual Doses for Common Gastrointestinal Medications

Most medications to treat GI conditions can be taken orally. Sometimes, as with antacids, the medication is available in a chewable form. This allows the patient to chew the tablet, drink water, and therefore suspend the medication in the stomach, allowing it to work quickly. Other times, antacids are available in liquid form, reducing the amount of water needed for effective use. Stomach ulcers can be of concern for hospitalized patients who may not be able to take medications by mouth; therefore, some medications used to treat and prevent ulcers can be given intravenously.

Some medications are best if applied more directly to the affected area. Rectal suppositories can be used, as can rectal liquids. These routes of administration may be used with medications to treat ulcerative colitis and constipation.

Common Side Effects of Gastrointestinal Medications

Gastrointestinal medications may have side effects related to the GI system. For instance, some medications that treat heartburn may cause an upset stomach, nausea, vomiting, and diarrhea. Fortunately, these side effects are not common; headache is the most common side effect with medications that treat GERD.

Laxatives and other medications used to treat constipation run the risk of causing diarrhea. Some medications used to treat ulcerative colitis may cause abdominal pain and nausea. Cardiovascular effects, such as an increased heart rate, can be present with some medications used to treat obesity.

Terminology and Common Abbreviations Used with Gastrointestinal Medications

See Table 2-1, page 13, for abbreviations.

What's in a Name?

Table 10-2. Examples of USAN Stems for Gastrointestinal Medications

Stem	Description	Example
-tidine	H2-receptor antagonists (cimetidine type)	famotidine
-vastatin	Antihyperlipidemics (HMG-CoA inhibitors)	atorvastatin
-setron	Serotonin 5-HT3 antagonists	ondansetron
-prazole	Antiulcer agents (benzimidazole derivatives)	omeprazole

Sample Prescription for Gastrointestinal Medications

DEA # BD0000000

John Doe, M.D.
123 Any Street
Any Town, Any State 00000
Tel. (123) 456-7890   Fax. (123) 456-1234

NAME _Jackie Trueman_

ADDRESS _1227 18th St._

℞   Adipex-P #30 (thirty)

Sig: T I T PO QD

_____ J. Doe, _____ M.D.
(Signature)

REFILL _Rfx2_

This prescription should be interpreted as Adipex-P (phentermine) 37.5mg, take one capsule by mouth daily. Dispense 30 capsules with two refills.

Technician Tip

Some states have restrictions on the use of weight loss medications. Restrictions could include the number of concurrent fills allowed, or they may require that a patient see his or her physician on a regular basis for monitoring. Check with your pharmacist if you are unsure of any specific regulations in your state for weight loss medications. ℞

Alternative Therapies for Gastrointestinal Conditions

Many alternative and home remedies exist for treating GI conditions. Clinicians often hesitate to recommend home remedies as first-line therapies, however. Nonetheless, many over-the-counter therapies exist to treat GI conditions so that home remedies are not the only option.

Additional nondrug therapies recommended by some clinicians include increasing fiber intake and regular physical activity to treat mild constipation. Modifying a patient's eating habits may treat heartburn and GERD. Some changes such as reducing spicy foods, fatty foods, caffeine, and alcohol can help reduce the symptoms of heartburn and GERD. Some of these approaches may be tried in addition to medication.

Chapter Summary !

Symptomatic control of several gastrointestinal system conditions can be important for patients.

℞ Nausea and vomiting may be related to several illnesses and conditions or may even be related to other medication use, such as chemotherapy for cancer treatment. Various treatments exist for different causes of nausea and vomiting

℞ Constipation and diarrhea can be frustrating for patients, and different routes of administration may exist for treatment

℞ Some medications are available for the treatment of obesity, although health professionals should pay close attention to legal restrictions on the use of medications for weight loss

℞ Heartburn and GERD are prevalent conditions that may require treatment. If symptoms are mild, OTC treatment may be appropriate, but it is always good for patients to tell their pharmacist and physician about any OTC treatments they are using

Although many oral medications are available to treat such conditions, other routes may be used if the patient has trouble taking medications orally. Because these conditions may be temporary, short-term therapy may be indicated, or chronic therapy may be necessary.

STUDENT NAME _____

DATE _____ INSTRUCTOR'S NAME _____

ANATOMY, PHYSIOLOGY, AND PHARMACOLOGY QUESTIONS

Identify whether the following questions are true or false (circle one).

1. Drugs such as orlistat can be used to prevent or heal GI damage caused by NSAIDS.
   TRUE   FALSE

2. Gastroesophageal reflux disease is the same as heartburn.
   TRUE   FALSE

3. Obesity can be treated by medications that help to reduce appetite.
   TRUE   FALSE

4. Constipation can be treated with laxatives or stool softeners.
   TRUE   FALSE

5. Nausea and vomiting can be caused by chemotherapy treatment for cancer.
   TRUE   FALSE

MEDICATION QUESTIONS:

Match the following brand-name products with their generic names.

1. _____ Lomotil
2. _____ MiraLAX
3. _____ Carafate
4. _____ Tums
5. _____ Alli
6. _____ Tagamet
7. _____ Nexium
8. _____ Cytotec

A. cimetidine
B. calcium carbonate
C. orlistat
D. misoprostol
E. esomeprazole
F. polyethylene glycol 3350
G. sucralfate
H. diphenoxylate and atropine

9. _____ Gas X

10. _____ Metamucil

11. _____ HalfLytely and bisacodyl

12. _____ Colace

13. _____ AcipHex

14. _____ Pepcid

15. _____ Mylanta

16. _____ Maalox

A. rabeprazole

B. simethicone

C. aluminum hydroxide, magnesium hydroxide, and simethicone

D. psyllium

E. aluminum hydroxide and magnesium hydroxide

F. famotidine

G. polyethylene glycol electrolyte solution and bisacodyl

H. docusate

17. _____ Protonix

18. _____ TriLyte

19. _____ Reglan

20. _____ Azulfidine

21. _____ Prevpac

22. _____ Imodium

23. _____ Helidac

24. _____ Asacol

A. polyethylene glycol electrolyte solution

B. mesalamine

C. pantoprazole

D. lansoprazole, amoxicillin, and clarithromycin

E. bismuth, metronidazole, and tetracycline

F. sulfasalazine

G. metoclopramide

H. loperamide

25. _____ Bentyl

26. _____ Compazine

27. _____ Phenergan

28. _____ Prilosec OTC

29. _____ Kaopectate

30. _____ Zofran

31. _____ Prevacid

32. _____ Axid

A. promethazine

B. prochlorperazine

C. attapulgite

D. nizatidine

E. lansoprazole

F. dicyclomine

G. omeprazole

H. ondansetron

STUDENT NAME _____

DATE _____ INSTRUCTOR'S NAME _____

33. _____ Zantac	A. granisetron
34. _____ Dulcolax	B. hyoscyamine
35. _____ Anaspaz	C. lactulose
36. _____ Enulose	D. bisacodyl
37. _____ Adipex-P	E. ranitidine
38. _____ Anzemet	F. phentermine
39. _____ Kytril	G. omeprazole
40. _____ Prilosec	H. dolasetron

41. _____ Imodium Multi-Symptom Relief	A. mesalamine
42. _____ Pentasa	B. hyoscyamine
43. _____ Octreotide	C. loperamide and simethicone
44. _____ Preparation H	D. polyethylene glycol electrolyte solution
45. _____ Levsin	E. calcium carbonate and magnesium hydroxide
46. _____ Kristalose	F. lactulose
47. _____ GoLYTELY	G. phenylephrine
48. _____ Rolaids	H. Sandostatin

Select a common and appropriate frequency of administration (circle one).

1. Xenical	q.d.	b.i.d.	t.i.d.	q.i.d.
2. Cytotec	q.d.	b.i.d.	t.i.d.	q.i.d.
3. Prilosec OTC	q.d.	b.i.d.	t.i.d.	q.i.d.
4. Reglan	q.d.	b.i.d.	t.i.d.	q.i.d.
5. Nexium	q.d.	b.i.d.	t.i.d.	q.i.d.
6. Prevpac	q.d.	b.i.d.	t.i.d.	q.i.d.
7. Metamucil	q.d.	b.i.d.	t.i.d.	q.i.d.
8. sucralfate	q.d.	b.i.d.	t.i.d.	q.i.d.
9. Bentyl	q.d.	b.i.d.	t.i.d.	q.i.d.
10. pantoprazole	q.d.	b.i.d.	t.i.d.	q.i.d.

Select the correct dosage form (circle one).

1.	Mylanta	Liquid	Tablet	Parenteral
2.	Dulcolax	Liquid	Tablet	Parenteral
3.	AcipHex	Liquid	Tablet	Parenteral
4.	Kristalose	Liquid	Tablet	Parenteral
5.	octreotide	Liquid	Tablet	Parenteral
6.	misoprostol	Liquid	Tablet	Parenteral
7.	Kaopectate	Liquid	Tablet	Parenteral
8.	Maalox	Liquid	Tablet	Parenteral
9.	Tums	Liquid	Tablet	Parenteral
10.	Rolaids	Liquid	Tablet	Parenteral

Identify whether the following are available parenterally, orally, or both (circle one).

1.	hyoscyamine	Parenteral	Oral	Both
2.	orlistat	Parenteral	Oral	Both
3.	psyllium	Parenteral	Oral	Both
4.	Anzemet	Parenteral	Oral	Both
5.	lactulose	Parenteral	Oral	Both
6.	Sandostatin	Parenteral	Oral	Both
7.	Sancuso	Parenteral	Oral	Both
8.	CoLyte	Parenteral	Oral	Both
9.	Protonix	Parenteral	Oral	Both
10.	Tums	Parenteral	Oral	Both

Identify whether the following are available OTC or are Rx only (circle one).

1.	Prevacid 24HR	OTC	Rx Only
2.	Tagamet-HB	OTC	Rx Only
3.	Nexium	OTC	Rx Only
4.	Zantac 75	OTC	Rx Only
5.	Zofran	OTC	Rx Only
6.	Axid-AR	OTC	Rx Only
7.	Prevpac	OTC	Rx Only
8.	Reglan	OTC	Rx Only
9.	Imodium AD	OTC	Rx Only
10.	Tums	OTC	Rx Only

STUDENT NAME _____

DATE _____ INSTRUCTOR'S NAME _____

Select the appropriate main use/drug class (circle one).

1. dolasetron	Heartburn	Diarrhea	Nausea
2. Maalox	Heartburn	Diarrhea	Nausea
3. famotidine	Heartburn	Diarrhea	Nausea
4. diphenoxylate and atropine	Heartburn	Diarrhea	Nausea
5. Zofran	Heartburn	Diarrhea	Nausea
6. Axid	Heartburn	Diarrhea	Nausea
7. Sancuso	Heartburn	Diarrhea	Nausea
8. Kaopectate	Heartburn	Diarrhea	Nausea
9. calcium carbonate	Heartburn	Diarrhea	Nausea
10. Imodium	Heartburn	Diarrhea	Nausea

Identify whether the following questions are true or false (circle one).

1. Chronulac is used to treat constipation.

   TRUE   FALSE

2. Rowasa is used to treat nausea.

   TRUE   FALSE

3. Dulcolax can be given as a suppository.

   TRUE   FALSE

4. Lactulose is used to treat diarrhea.

   TRUE   FALSE

5. Imodium Multi-Symptom Relief can be used to treat nausea.

   TRUE   FALSE

6. Kaopectate is a brand name of attapulgite.

   TRUE   FALSE

7. Rabeprazole can be used to treat gastrointestinal reflux.

   TRUE   FALSE

8. Phenergan can be given PO, IV, IM, or rectally.

   TRUE   FALSE

9. Compazine is used to treat constipation.

   TRUE   FALSE

10. Cytotec is used to treat diarrhea.

   TRUE   FALSE

Select a common strength for the following medications.

1. misoprostol
   a. 25mcg
   b. 50mcg
   c. 75mcg
   d. 100mcg

2. orlistat
   a. 61mg
   b. 75mg
   c. 100mg
   d. 150mg

3. omeprazole
   a. 5mg
   b. 10mg
   c. 15mg
   d. 20mg

4. Dulcolax
   a. 1mg
   b. 2mg
   c. 4mg
   d. 5mg

5. Zantac
   a. 15mg
   b. 150mg
   c. 1000mg
   d. 1500mg

6. Protonix
   a. 40mg
   b. 50mg
   c. 60mg
   d. 75mg

7. sulfasalazine
   a. 100mg
   b. 200mg
   c. 500mg
   d. 1000mg

8. Adipex-P
   a. 30mg
   b. 60mg
   c. 90mg
   d. 120mg

9. dexlansoprazole
   a. 10mg
   b. 20mg
   c. 30mg
   d. 40mg

10. prochlorperazine
    a. 1mg
    b. 10mg
    c. 100mg
    d. 1000mg

11. nizatidine
    a. 300mg
    b. 400mg
    c. 500mg
    d. 600mg

12. cimetidine
    a. 100mg
    b. 200mg
    c. 500mg
    d. 1000mg

13. calcium carbonate
    a. 100mg
    b. 500mg
    c. 1500mg
    d. 2500mg

14. docusate
    a. 50mg
    b. 60mg
    c. 70mg
    d. 80mg

15. esomeprazole
    a. 5mg
    b. 10mg
    c. 40mg
    d. 80mg

STUDENT NAME _____

DATE _____   INSTRUCTOR'S NAME _____

Select the best available answer for the following questions.

1. Chronulac and Enulose are both brand names for _____.

   a. docusate
   b. lactulose
   c. pantoprazole
   d. omeprazole

2. Compazine can be given _____.

   a. intravenously
   b. rectally
   c. intramuscularly
   d. subcutaneously

3. The generic name for Dulcolax is _____ and it is used as a _____.

   a. mesalamine, treatment for ulcerative colitis
   b. lactulose, laxative
   c. bisacodyl, laxative
   d. sulfasalazine, treatment for ulcerative colitis

4. Ondansetron is generic for _____.

   a. Zofran
   b. Kytril
   c. Anzemet
   d. Metamucil

5. Preparation H is a drug that is used to _____.

   a. treat gastroesophageal reflux
   b. treat diarrhea
   c. treat hemorrhoids
   d. treat ulcers

6. Adipex-P is used to treat _____.

   a. hemorrhoids
   b. diarrhea
   c. obesity
   d. ulcerative colitis

7. What do ranitidine and Axid have in common? _____.

   a. Both are used to treat diarrhea
   b. Both are given intravenously
   c. Both are used to treat heartburn
   d. Both are given intramuscularly

8. Rolaids contain _____.

    a. aluminum hydroxide and magnesium hydroxide
    b. aluminum hydroxide, magnesium hydroxide, and simethicone
    c. bismuth, metronidazole, and tetracycline
    d. calcium carbonate and magnesium hydroxide

9. The proper route of administration of Gas-X is _____ and its generic name is _____.

    a. PO, simethicone
    b. PO, psyllium
    c. IV, simethicone
    d. IV, psyllium

10. Lansoprazole is used to _____.

    a. treat diarrhea
    b. treat ulcers
    c. treat ulcerative colitis
    d. treat obesity

11. Levbid and NuLev both contain _____.

    a. mesalamine
    b. phentermine
    c. hyoscyamine
    d. sulfasalazine

12. The generic name of Bentyl is _____.

    a. mesalamine
    b. sibutramine
    c. dicyclomine
    d. metoclopramide

13. Nexium can be given _____.

    a. IV
    b. IM
    c. SQ
    d. IN

14. Prevpac contains _____.

    a. bismuth, metronidazole, and tetracycline
    b. lansoprazole, amoxicillin, and clarithromycin
    c. calcium carbonate and magnesium hydroxide
    d. aluminum hydroxide, magnesium hydroxide, and simethicone

15. Calcium carbonate is generic for _____.

    a. Prilosec
    b. Helidac
    c. Protonix
    d. Tums

STUDENT NAME _____

DATE _____   INSTRUCTOR'S NAME _____

DISCUSSION AND CRITICAL THINKING QUESTIONS

1. Why would a patient take antacids in addition to a medication such as ranitidine?

2. What restrictions exist in your state for the use of medications to treat weight loss?

3. Which categories of gastrointestinal medications could logically be taken PRN, and which should be scheduled?

4. Should patients tell their doctor or pharmacist if they are taking OTC medications? Why or why not?

_____

_____

_____

_____

_____

5. What lifestyle changes can patients make to help treat obesity?

_____

_____

_____

_____

_____

_____

STUDENT NAME _____

DATE _____ INSTRUCTOR'S NAME _____

SAMPLE PRESCRIPTIONS

DEA # BD0000000

John Doe, M.D.
123 Any Street
Any Town, Any State 00000
Tel. (123) 456-7890   Fax. (123) 456-1234

NAME _Katie McPeek_____

ADDRESS _845 S. Perry St._____

Rx   Lomotil 2.5mg/0.025mg
             #12 (twelve)

Sig: T 1 T QID PRN

_____ J. Doe, _____ M.D.
                  (Signature)

REFILL _NR_____

NDC 0025-0061-31
100 Tablets   **Rx only**
Lomotil® ©
(diphenoxylate
hydrochloride and
atropine sulfate tablets USP)

2.5 mg/0.025 mg*

Distributed by
Pfizer G.D. Searle LLC
Division of Pfizer Inc, NY, NY 10017

1. What is the generic name for Lomotil?

_____

_____

2. How would you translate the Sig code into plain English so that the patient could understand the directions for use?

_____

_____

_____

3. How many refills are given on this prescription?

_____

_____

_____

4. What common condition(s) does this medication treat?

_____

_____

_____

5. What other dosage forms are available for this medication?

_____

_____

_____

6. What is the days supply of this medication?

_____

_____

_____

7. What schedule is this medication?

_____

_____

_____

8. What is the maximum number of refills allowed on this prescription and why?

_____

_____

_____

STUDENT NAME _____

DATE _____ INSTRUCTOR'S NAME _____

DEA # BD0000000

John Doe, M.D.
123 Any Street
Any Town, Any State 00000
Tel. (123) 456-7890   Fax. (123) 456-1234

NAME   _Stewart Lockman_____

ADDRESS   _132 Maple St._____

Rx   Xenical 120mg #90

Sig: T 1 T PO TID AC

_____ J. Doe, _____ M.D.
(Signature)

REFILL   _Rfx 1_____

---

1. What is the generic name for Xenical?

   _____

   _____

2. How would you translate the Sig code into plain English so that the patient could understand the directions for use?

   _____

   _____

   _____

3. How many refills are given on this prescription?

_____

_____

_____

_____

4. What is a common use for this medication?

_____

_____

_____

_____

_____

5. What is the days supply for this medication?

_____

_____

_____

_____

_____

6. What is the brand name of the over-the-counter product with the same active ingredient?

_____

_____

_____

_____

_____

STUDENT NAME _____

DATE _____ INSTRUCTOR'S NAME _____

DEA # BD0000000

John Doe, M.D.
123 Any Street
Any Town, Any State 00000
Tel. (123) 456-7890   Fax. (123) 456-1234

NAME   _Darryl Candle_____

ADDRESS   _922 Louisville Ct._____

Rx   GoLYTELY #1 container

Sig: T 8oz PO Q10min until gone

_____ J. Doe, _____ M.D.
                         (Signature)

REFILL   _NR_____

---

1. What is the generic name for GoLYTELY?

   _____

   _____

2. How would you translate the directions from the Sig code into plain English so that the patient could understand the directions for use?

   _____

   _____

   _____

3. How many refills are given on this prescription?

4. What is a common use for this medication?

5. How many 8oz doses are required to take the entire quantity?

Urinary and Reproductive Medications

11

KEY TERMS

Anabolic steroids

Antimuscarinic

Erectile dysfunction (ED)

Estrogen

Hormone

Impotence

Menopause

Oral contraceptives

Ovaries

Progestin

Testes

Testosterone

LEARNING OBJECTIVES

After completing this chapter, the student will be able to:

1. Describe the basic anatomy and physiology of the urinary and reproductive systems

2. Explain the therapeutic effects of common medications used to treat diseases of the urinary and reproductive systems

3. List the brand and generic names of common medications used to treat diseases of the urinary and reproductive systems

4. Identify available dosage forms for common urinary and reproductive system medications

5. Identify routes of administration for common urinary and reproductive system medications

6. Identify usual doses for common urinary and reproductive system medications

7. List common side effects of frequently prescribed urinary and reproductive system medications

8. Define medical terms commonly used when treating diseases of the urinary and reproductive systems

9. List abbreviations for terms associated with the use of medication therapy for common diseases affecting the urinary and reproductive systems

10. Describe alternative therapies commonly used to treat diseases of the urinary and reproductive systems

Basic Anatomy and Physiology of the Urinary System and the Reproductive System

The urinary system performs important functions in the body. Some of the many functions of the urinary system are the following: removal of waste products, maintaining fluid balance, and maintaining electrolyte and acid-base balances. The organs of the urinary system are shown in Figure 11-1 and include the kidney and urinary bladder.

The reproductive systems are different for males and females and have functions that provide for producing offspring. The main organs of the reproductive system in females are the ovaries, and in males they are the testes. See Figure 11-2 for a posterior view of the female reproductive organs. Female reproductive parts shown include ovary, uterine (fallopian) tube, ovarian ligament, round ligament, wall of uterus (endometrium, myometrium, perimetrium), cervical canal, cervical os, vagina, cervix, body of uterus, broad ligament (mesosalpinx, mesovarium, mesometrium), ovarian blood vessels, and suspensory ligament of ovary.

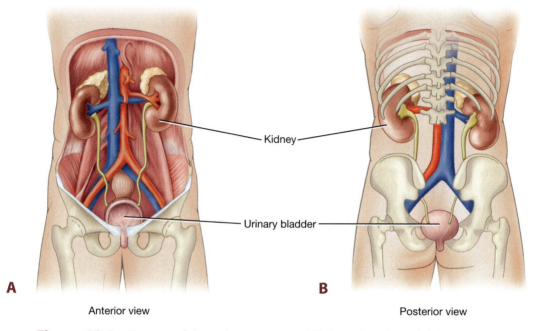

A — Anterior view

B — Posterior view

Figure 11-1. Organs of the urinary system: (**A**) Anterior view; (**B**) Posterior view.

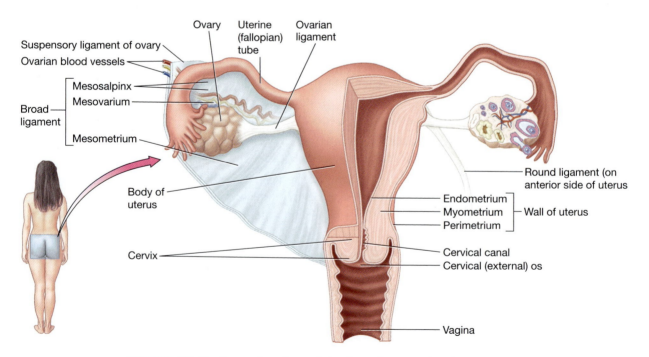

Figure 11-2. Posterior view of the female reproductive organs.

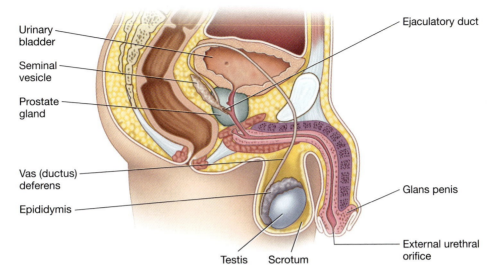

Figure 11-3. Parts of male urinary and reproductive system.

Parts of the male urinary and reproductive system are shown in Figure 11-3 and include the ejaculatory duct, glans penis, external urethral orifice, scrotum, testis, epididymis, vas deferens, prostate gland, seminal vesicle, and urinary bladder.

Knowing the following terms will be helpful as you learn about the medications used to treat conditions affecting the urinary and reproductive systems.

Anabolic steroids: Hormones that are derivatives of testosterone

Antimuscarinic: Effects associated with slowed heart rate, increased secretion by some glands, and increased activity of certain muscles, including those of the small intestine and bladder

Erectile dysfunction (ED): Condition in males associated with a failure to have or maintain an erection (impotence)

Estrogen: Hormone associated with the female reproductive system

Hormone: Chemicals in the body that are secreted by glands and circulate in the blood to have effects throughout the body

Impotence: Condition in males associated with a failure to have or maintain an erection (erectile dysfunction)

Menopause: Time in women when the natural cessation of menstruation occurs

Oral contraceptives: Medications that usually contain a combination of a progestin and an estrogen, but sometimes only a progestin, that prevent pregnancy

Ovaries: Female reproductive glands

Progestin: Hormone associated with the female reproductive system

Testes: Male reproductive glands

Testosterone: Hormone associated with the male reproductive system

Primer on Pharmacologic Actions of Urinary and Reproductive System Medications

The most common reproductive system agents are associated with hormone therapy. For females, two main categories of hormones are commonly prescribed: progestins, such as medroxyprogesterone (Provera), and estrogens, such as the conjugated estrogens (Premarin). For males, the common hormones prescribed are testosterone and derivatives of testosterone, such as stanozolol that are commonly known as anabolic steroids.

Progestins, such as medroxyprogesterone, are most commonly used to treat abnormal vaginal bleeding and can also be used to prevent overgrowth of the lining of the uterus. Progestins also trigger the uterus to produce other hormones. Progestins are a common component of many oral contraceptives.

Estrogens can be prescribed for a number of conditions associated with the regulation of hormonal balance. One example is to treat hot flashes in menopausal women; another is to supplement estrogen in premenopausal women to address conditions of low estrogen. Additionally, some estrogen products can be used to treat symptoms of certain types of breast and prostate cancers. Estrogens are also a common component of many oral contraceptives.

Testosterone is a hormone that is sometimes prescribed to treat the symptoms of low testosterone in men. Testosterone has effects on the growth, development, and functioning of the male sexual organs and typical male characteristics such as muscular build and deep voice.

Sildenafil (Viagra) is medication used to treat male impotence (erectile dysfunction). Sildenafil is not a hormone and is in a class of medications called phosphodiesterase (PDE) inhibitors. PDE inhibitors produce their effects by increasing blood flow to the penis during sexual stimulation.

Enlarged prostate glands are common in men over age 50. The condition of enlarged prostate is commonly known as benign prostatic hyperplasia (BPH). Symptoms of BPH include urinary hesitation, dribbling, urgency, and incomplete bladder emptying. Tamsulosin (Flomax) is an example of an alpha-blocker

that is sometimes used to treat BPH and works by relaxing muscles in the prostate and bladder. Finasteride (Proscar) is another type of drug used to treat BPH. Finasteride is an example of a 5-alpha reductase inhibitor and works by blocking the formation of a substance in the body that causes the prostate to enlarge.

The common urinary system medications are used to relieve urinary difficulties or treat painful urination. Tolterodine (Detrol) is a medication in the class antimuscarinics. Antimuscarinic agents prevent bladder contraction and are used to treat frequent urination, as well as inability to control urination. Phenazopyridine (Pyridium) is a medication used to treat painful urination commonly associated with urinary tract infections (UTIs), surgery, or examination procedures. Phenazopyridine has a analgesic effect on the urinary tract, but it does not cure infections (Table 11-1 and Table 11-2).

Table 11-1. Common Urinary and Reproductive Agents and Their Uses

Generic Name	Brand Name	Dosage Form	Route	Common Use	Common Frequency	Common Strengths
etonogestrel and ethinyl estradiol vaginal ring	NuvaRing	Ring	Intravaginally	Contraception	Insert ring for three weeks, remove ring for one week	0.12–0.015mg/24 hours
medroxyprogesterone injection	Depo-Provera	Parenteral	IM	Contraception	q.3months	150mg/ml
norelgestromin and ethinyl estradiol transdermal system	Ortho Evra Patch	Patch	Transdermally	Contraception	Apply patch for three weeks, remove patch for one week	150/20mcg/24 hours
sildenafil	Viagra	Tablet	PO	Erectile dysfunction	PRN	25mg, 50mg, 100mg
tadalafil	Cialis	Tablet	PO	Erectile dysfunction	PRN	5mg, 10mg, 20mg
vardenafil	Levitra	Tablet	PO	Erectile dysfunction	PRN	2.5mg, 5mg, 10mg, 20mg
conjugated equine estrogens	Premarin	Tablet	PO	Hormone replacement	q.d.	0.3mg, 0.45mg, 0.625mg, 0.9mg, 1.25mg
conjugated equine estrogens	Premarin Vaginal Cream	Cream	Intravaginally	Hormone replacement	q.d.×3 weeks, 1 week off	0.625mg/g

(Continued)

Table 11-1. Common Urinary and Reproductive Agents and Their Uses (Continued)

Generic Name	Brand Name	Dosage Form	Route	Common Use	Common Frequency	Common Strengths
conjugated equine estrogens, medroxyprogesterone	Premphase	Tablet	PO	Hormone replacement	q.d.	0.625mg, 0.625mg/5mg
conjugated equine estrogens, medroxyprogesterone	Prempro	Tablet	PO	Hormone replacement	q.d.	0.3mg/1.5mg, 0.45mg/1.5mg, 0.625mg/2.5mg, 0.625mg/5mg
esterified estrogens	Menest	Tablet	PO	Hormone replacement	q.d.×3 weeks, 1 week off	0.3mg, 0.625mg, 1.25mg, 2.5mg
estradiol	Estrace Vaginal Cream	Cream	Intravaginally	Hormone replacement	q.d.	0.1mg/g
estradiol	Estring Vaginal Ring	Ring	Intravaginally	Hormone replacement	Apply q.90days	2mg
estradiol	Alora	Patch	Transdermally	Hormone replacement	Apply twice weekly	0.025mg/24hr, 0.05mg/24hr, 0.075mg/24hr, 0.1 mg/24hr
estradiol	Climara	Patch	Transdermally	Hormone replacement	Apply once weekly	0.025mg/24hr, 0.0375mg/hr, 0.05mg/24hr, 0.06mg/hr, 0.075mg/24hr, 0.1 mg/24hr
estradiol	Estraderm	Patch	Transdermally	Hormone replacement	Apply twice weekly	0.05mg/24hr, 0.1 mg/24hr
estradiol	Vivelle Dot	Patch	Transdermally	Hormone replacement	Apply twice weekly	0.025mg/24hr, 0.0375mg/hr, 0.05mg/24hr, 0.075mg/24hr, 0.1 mg/24hr
estradiol	Vagifem	Tablet	Intravaginally	Hormone replacement	q.d., twice weekly	10mg, 25mg
estradiol, norethindrone	Activella	Tablet	PO	Hormone replacement	q.d.	0.5mg/0.1mg, 1mg/0.5mg
estradiol, norethindrone	Combipatch	Patch	Transdermally	Hormone replacement	Apply twice weekly	0.05mg/0.14mg, 0.05mg/0.25mg
estradiol, norgestimate	Ortho-Prefest	Tablet	PO	Hormone replacement	q.d.	1mg, 1mg/0.09mg
estropipate	Ortho-Est	Tablet	PO	Hormone replacement	q.d.	0.625mg

(Continued)

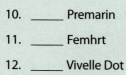

11. EXERCISES

9. _____ Cialis

10. _____ Premarin

11. _____ Femhrt

12. _____ Vivelle Dot

13. _____ Levitra

14. _____ Ortho-Est

15. _____ Ortho-Prefest

16. _____ Uroxatral

A. estradiol

B. conjugated equine estrogens

C. tadalafil

D. estradiol and norgestimate

E. ethinyl estradiol and norethindrone

F. alfuzosin

G. estropipate

H. vardenafil

17. _____ Enablex

18. _____ AndroGel

19. _____ Estrace

20. _____ Premphase

21. _____ Vesicare

22. _____ Activella

23. _____ Azo-Standard

24. _____ Climara

A. estradiol

B. solifenacin

C. testosterone

D. darifenacin

E. estradiol and norethindrone

F. micronized estradiol

G. phenazopyridine

H. conjugated equine estrogens and medroxyprogesterone

25. _____ Ditropan

26. _____ Cenestin

27. _____ Viagra

28. _____ Alora

29. _____ Pyridium

30. _____ Detrol LA

31. _____ Prempro

32. _____ Testim

A. conjugated equine estrogens and medroxyprogesterone

B. estradiol

C. tolterodine

D. phenazopyridine

E. testosterone

F. sildenafil

G. synthetic conjugated estrogen

H. oxybutynin

STUDENT NAME _____

DATE _____ INSTRUCTOR'S NAME _____

33. _____ Hytrin

34. _____ Cardura

35. _____ Flomax

36. _____ Depo-Testosterone

37. _____ Proscar

38. _____ Vagifem

39. _____ Avodart

A. dutasteride

B. estradiol

C. doxazosin

D. finasteride

E. testosterone

F. terazosin

G. tamsulosin

40. _____ Yasmin

41. _____ Modicon

42. _____ Desogen

43. _____ Ortho Micronor

44. _____ Demulen

45. _____ Nordette

46. _____ Low-Ogestrel

47. _____ Ortho-Tri-Cyclen

A. Cryselle

B. Ocella

C. Zovia

D. Errin

E. Apri

F. Necon

G. Portia

H. Tri-Sprintec

48. _____ Ortho Novum

49. _____ Ortho-Cyclen

50. _____ Alesse

51. _____ Seasonique

52. _____ Mircette

53. _____ Loestrin Fe

54. _____ Cyclessa

55. _____ Ovcon 35

A. Junel Fe

B. Quasense

C. Kariva

D. Velivet

E. Nortrel 7/7/7

F. Balziva

G. Aviane

H. Sprintec

56. _____ Trivora   A. Portia

57. _____ Brevicon   B. Enpresse

58. _____ Low-Ogestrel   C. MonoNessa

59. _____ Estrostep Fe   D. Tri-Legest Fe

60. _____ Nordette   E. Lo/Ovral

61. _____ Ortho-Cyclen   F. Jolessa

62. _____ Seasonale   G. Nortrel

Select a common and appropriate schedule administration (circle one).

1.	Menest	q.d.	q.d.×3 weeks, 1 week off
2.	Premarin	q.d.	q.d.×3 weeks, 1 week off
3.	Estrace	q.d.	q.d.×3 weeks, 1 week off
4.	Premarin vaginal cream	q.d.	q.d.×3 weeks, 1 week off
5.	Provera	q.d.	q.d.×3 weeks, 1 week off
6.	Alora	Once weekly	Twice weekly
7.	Combipatch	Once weekly	Twice weekly
8.	Climara	Once weekly	Twice weekly
9.	Estraderm	Once weekly	Twice weekly
10.	Vivelle Dot	Once weekly	Twice weekly

Select the correct route of administration (circle one).

1.	Estraderm	PO	Transdermally	Intravaginally
2.	Activella	PO	Transdermally	Intravaginally
3.	NuvaRing	PO	Transdermally	Intravaginally
4.	Detrol	PO	Transdermally	Intravaginally
5.	Vagifem	PO	Transdermally	Intravaginally
6.	VESIcare	PO	Transdermally	Intravaginally
7.	Estring vaginal ring	PO	Transdermally	Intravaginally
8.	Climara	PO	Transdermally	Intravaginally
9.	Vivelle Dot	PO	Transdermally	Intravaginally
10.	Femhrt	PO	Transdermally	Intravaginally

STUDENT NAME _____

DATE _____ INSTRUCTOR'S NAME _____

Select the appropriate main use/drug class (circle one).

1.	Ortho Evra	Contraception	Hormone replacement
2.	Combipatch	Contraception	Hormone replacement
3.	Climara	Contraception	Hormone replacement
4.	Depo-Provera	Contraception	Hormone replacement
5.	Premphase	Contraception	Hormone replacement
6.	NuvaRing	Contraception	Hormone replacement
7.	Ortho-Est	Contraception	Hormone replacement
8.	Cenestin	Contraception	Hormone replacementr
9.	Trivora	Contraception	Hormone replacement
10.	Yasmin	Contraception	Hormone replacement

Identify whether the following questions are true or false (circle one).

1. AndroGel is a hormone replacement product that is applied topically.

   TRUE   FALSE

2. Azo-Standard is a urinary tract analgesic.

   TRUE   FALSE

3. Vardenafil is commonly given parenterally.

   TRUE   FALSE

4. Alfuzosin is used to treat BPH.

   TRUE   FALSE

5. Depo-Testosterone is given every week.

   TRUE   FALSE

6. Enablex is a hormone replacement.

   TRUE   FALSE

7. Estraderm, Vivelle Dot, and Climara are all patches.

   TRUE   FALSE

8. Tadalafil is primarily used to treat urinary incontinence.

   TRUE   FALSE

9. Oxybutynin must be dosed q.i.d.

   TRUE   FALSE

10. Depo-Provera is given parentally every 3 months.

   TRUE   FALSE

Select a common strength for the following medications.

1. Detrol LA
   a. 0.5mg
   b. 4mg
   c. 10mg
   d. 50mg

2. Ortho-Est
   a. 0.625mg
   b. 0.75mg
   c. 0.875mg
   d. 1mg

3. Estrace
   a. 0.1mg
   b. 0.625mg
   c. 0.9mg
   d. 2mg

4. Depo-Provera
   a. 100mg/ml
   b. 150mg/ml
   c. 500mg/ml
   d. 5000mg/ml

5. Provera
   a. 1mg
   b. 5mg
   c. 25mg
   d. 100mg

6. Prempro
   a. 0.625mg/2.5mg
   b. 1mg/1.5mg
   c. 5mg/5mg
   d. 10mg/2.5mg

7. sildenafil
   a. 20mg
   b. 30mg
   c. 40mg
   d. 50mg

8. finasteride
   a. 5mg
   b. 10mg
   c. 15mg
   d. 20mg

9. Cialis
   a. 1mg
   b. 10mg
   c. 100mg
   d. 1000mg

10. Flomax
   a. 0.1mg
   b. 0.4mg
   c. 1mg
   d. 4mg

11. Vagifem
   a. 1mg
   b. 5mg
   c. 15mg
   d. 25mg

12. Avodart
   a. 0.5mg
   b. 1mg
   c. 1.5mg
   d. 2mg

13. Enablex
   a. 10mg
   b. 15mg
   c. 20mg
   d. 25mg

14. Menest
   a. 0.5mg
   b. 0.625mg
   c. 1mg
   d. 2mg

15. terazosin
   a. 4mg
   b. 5mg
   c. 6mg
   d. 7mg

STUDENT NAME _____

DATE _____ INSTRUCTOR'S NAME _____

Select the best available answer for the following questions.

1. Cyclessa is considered _____.

   a. a treatment for benign prostatic hyperplasia
   b. an oral contraceptive
   c. a urinary tract analgesic
   d. a treatment for urinary incontinence

2. Ditropan XL is a drug that is used to _____.

   a. treat urinary tract pain
   b. treat erectile dysfunction
   c. provide hormone replacement
   d. treat urinary incontinence

3. The generic name for Pyridium is _____, and it is used as a _____.

   a. solifenacin, treatment for overactive bladder
   b. phenazopyridine, treatment for overactive bladder
   c. solifenacin, urinary tract analgesic
   d. phenazopyridine, urinary tract analgesic

4. Doxazosin is generic for _____.

   a. Cardura
   b. Proscar
   c. Hytrin
   d. Flomax

5. Premarin is used as a(n) _____.

   a. a hormone replacement
   b. an oral contraceptive
   c. a treatment for enlarged prostate
   d. a urinary tract analgesic

6. Prempro contains _____.

   a. tolterodine
   b. norelgestromin and ethinyl estradiol
   c. tadalafil
   d. conjugated equine estrogens and medroxyprogesterone.

7. The proper route of administration of NuvaRing is _____, and its generic name is _____.

   a. Intravaginally, etonogestrel and ethinyl estradiol
   b. PO, etonogestrel and ethinyl estradiol
   c. Intravaginally, medroxyprogesterone
   d. PO, medroxyprogesterone

8. Estrace and Estraderm are both brand names for _____.

    a. medroxyprogesterone
    b. estradiol
    c. synthetic conjugated estrogens
    d. norgestimate

9. What do Combipatch and Ortho Evra have in common? _____

    a. Both are patches
    b. Both are tablets
    c. Both are given parenterally
    d. Both are creams

10. Trivora is considered _____.

    a. an oral contraceptive
    b. a treatment for benign prostatic hyperplasia
    c. a urinary tract analgesic
    d. a treatment for urinary incontinence

11. The generic name of Avodart is _____.

    a. vardenafil
    b. darifenacin
    c. dutasteride
    d. solifenacin

12. Flomax is used to _____.

    a. replace hormones
    b. treat benign prostatic hyperplasia
    c. treat an overactive bladder
    d. treat urinary tract pain

13. Provera contains _____.

    a. estradiol
    b. medroxyprogesterone
    c. estropipate
    d. conjugated equine estrogens

14. Tolterodine is generic for _____.

    a. Detrol
    b. Ditropan
    c. Levitra
    d. Cialis

15. Testim is available as a _____.

    a. patch
    b. tablet
    c. gel
    d. ring

STUDENT NAME _____

DATE _____ INSTRUCTOR'S NAME _____

DISCUSSION AND CRITICAL THINKING QUESTIONS

1. What are the advantages and disadvantages of hormone patches?

   _____
   _____
   _____
   _____
   _____

2. Does your pharmacy stock over-the-counter products for contraception? What types are available?

   _____
   _____
   _____
   _____
   _____

3. Many oral contraceptives work best if taken regularly, even at the same time each day. What drug options exist that may be easier for women who have a hard time taking a pill regularly?

   _____
   _____
   _____
   _____
   _____

4. Some oral contraceptives change a woman's menstrual cycle so that she only has a period every three months. Why might this be good or bad for some women?

5. What is the difference between benign prostatic hyperplasia and prostate cancer?

STUDENT NAME _____

DATE _____ INSTRUCTOR'S NAME _____

SAMPLE PRESCRIPTIONS

DEA # BD0000000

John Doe, M.D.
123 Any Street
Any Town, Any State 00000
Tel. (123) 456-7890   Fax. (123) 456-1234

NAME _Evelyn Mathison_____

ADDRESS _1993 Courtney Ln._____

Rx   Detrol LA 4mg #90

Sig: T 1 T PO QD

_____ J. Doe, M.D.
(Signature)

REFILL _Rfx3_____

1. What is the generic name for Detrol?

   _____

   _____

2. How would you translate the Sig code into plain English so that the patient could understand the directions for use?

   _____

   _____

   _____

3. How many refills are given on this prescription?

_____

_____

_____

_____

4. What common condition(s) does this medication treat?

_____

_____

_____

_____

5. What is the days supply for this medication?

_____

_____

_____

_____

11. EXERCISES

STUDENT NAME _____

DATE _____ INSTRUCTOR'S NAME _____

DEA # BD0000000

John Doe, M.D.
123 Any Street
Any Town, Any State 00000
Tel. (123) 456-7890   Fax. (123) 456-1234

NAME *Daniel McCoy*

ADDRESS *1472 Columbus Ave.*

Rx   *Cialis 20mg #10*

Sig: *T 1 T PO QD PRN*

_____ *J. Doe,*   M.D.
                    (Signature)

REFILL *Rfx1*

NDC 0002-4464-30
30 Tablets

Cialis
(tadalafil) tablets
20mg

Rx only   *Lilly*

www.cialis.com
Eli Lilly and Company
Indianapolis, IN 46285, USA

---

1. What is the generic name for Cialis?

_____

_____

2. How would you translate the Sig code into plain English so that the patient could understand the directions for use?

_____

_____

_____

3. How many refills are given on this prescription?

4. What other common strengths are available for Cialis oral tablets?

5. What is a common use for this medication?

STUDENT NAME _____

DATE _____ INSTRUCTOR'S NAME _____

DEA # BD0000000

John Doe, M.D.
123 Any Street
Any Town, Any State 00000
Tel. (123) 456-7890   Fax. (123) 456-1234

NAME _Britney Hill_____

ADDRESS _822 Sylvania Ln._____

Rx   Nuvaring #1

Sig: Insert 1 ring vaginally x 3 weeks
        Remove x 1 week

_____J. Doe,_____ M.D.
          (Signature)

REFILL _RFx5_____

1. What is the generic name for Nuvaring?

   _____

   _____

2. How would you translate the Sig code into plain English so that the patient could understand the directions for use?

   _____

   _____

   _____

3. How many refills are given on this prescription?

_____

_____

_____

_____

4. What is a common use for this medication?

_____

_____

_____

_____

Eye, Ear, Nose, Mouth, and Throat Medications

12

KEY TERMS

Ocular

Ophthalmic

Otic

LEARNING OBJECTIVES

After completing this chapter, the student will be able to:

1. Describe the basic anatomy and physiology of the eye, ear, nose, mouth, and throat

2. Explain the therapeutic effects of common medications used to treat diseases of the eye, ear, nose, mouth, and throat

3. List the brand and generic names of common medications used to treat diseases of the eye, ear, nose, mouth and throat

4. Identify available dosage forms for common eye, ear, nose, and throat medications

5. Identify routes of administration for common eye, ear, nose, and throat medications

6. Identify usual doses for common eye, ear, nose, and throat medications

7. List common side effects of frequently prescribed eye, ear, nose, and throat medications

8. Define medical terms commonly used when treating diseases of eyes, ears, nose, and throat

9. List abbreviations for terms associated with use of medication therapy for common diseases affecting the eyes, ears, nose, mouth, and throat

10. Describe alternative therapies commonly used to treat diseases of the eyes, ears, nose, mouth and throat

Basic Anatomy and Physiology of the Eyes, Ears, Nose, Mouth, and Throat

The eyes, ears, nose, mouth, and throat are parts of the body associated with sensory perception. The eye is the organ associated with the sense of vision; the ear is the organ associated with the sense of hearing; the nose is the organ associated with the sense of smell; and the throat is part of the oral cavity and includes organs associated with taste perception.

The eyeball is a hollow organ surrounded by muscles and accessory structures. Figure 12-1 shows external and accessory structures of the eye, and Figure 12-2 shows the muscles surrounding the eye.

The ear contains components for both hearing and equilibrium. Figure 12-3 shows the anatomy of the ear and the parts that make up the outer, middle, and inner ear.

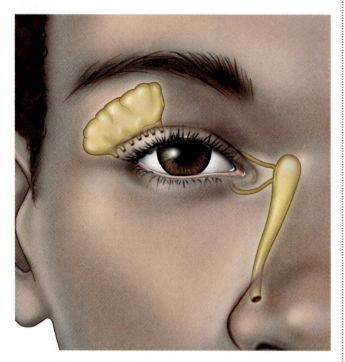

Figure 12-1. External and accessory structures of the eye.

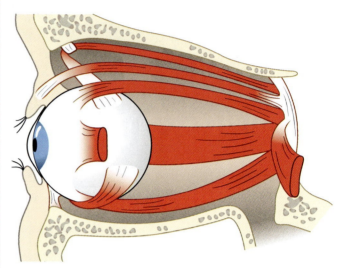

Figure 12-2. Muscles surrounding the eye.

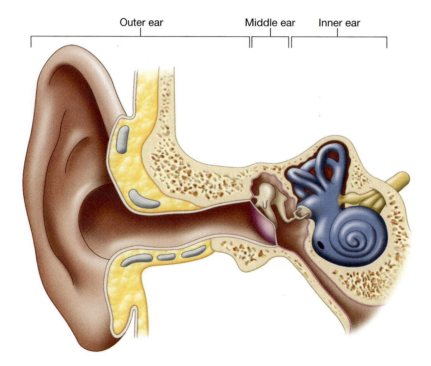

Figure 12-3. The anatomy of the ear.

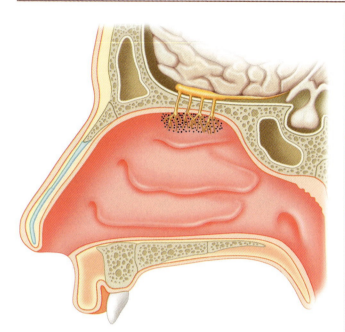

Figure 12-4. The nasal cavity.

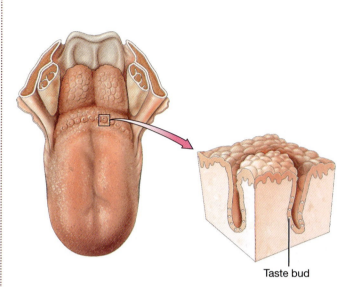

Taste bud

Figure 12-5. The surface of the tongue.

The senses of smell and taste are associated with the nose and mouth. Figure 12-4 shows the nasal cavity. Figure 12-5 shows the surface of the tongue, including the taste buds, that are important for taste perception. The nose also functions as part of the respiratory system (see Chapter 9), and the mouth and throat have important functions in the digestive system (see Chapter 10).

Knowing the following terms will be helpful as you learn about the medications used to treat conditions affecting the eyes, ears, nose, mouth, and throat.

Ocular: Pertaining to the eye
Ophthalmic: Pertaining to the eye
Otic: Pertaining to the ear

Primer on Pharmacologic Actions of Eye, Ear, Nose, Mouth, and Throat Agents

Ophthalmic agents are those used to treat conditions of the eye. The most common types of ophthalmic agents are associated with infections, glaucoma, allergies, and inflammation. Ocular anti-infective agents work in the same ways as other anti-infective agents; the preparations or dosage forms are specifically designed for application directly to the eye.

Otic agents are used to treat conditions of the ear. The most common types of otic agents are associated with infections, pain, and earwax buildup.

Agents used to treat conditions of the nose have effects on the respiratory system and were presented in Chapter 9 of this workbook.

Agents used to treat conditions of the mouth and throat include dental hygiene products as well as sore throat remedies (Table 12-1).

Table 12-1. Common Eyes, Ears, Nose, and Throat Agents and Their Uses

Generic Name	Brand Name	Dosage Form	Route	Common Use	Common Frequency	Common Strengths
beclomethasone	Beconase	Nasal spray	IN	Allergies, anti-inflammatory	b.i.d.	168mcg
ciclesonide	Omnaris	Nasal spray	IN	Allergies, anti-inflammatory	q.d.	50mg
cromolyn (OTC)	NasalCrom	Nasal spray	IN	Allergies	t.i.d.–q.i.d.	40mg
fluticasone	Veramyst, Flonase	Nasal spray	IN	Allergies, anti-inflammatory	q.d.	27.5mcg, 50mcg
mometasone	Nasonex	Nasal spray	IN	Allergies, anti-inflammatory	q.d.	50mcg
triamcinolone	Nasacort	Nasal spray	IN	Allergies, anti-inflammatory	q.d.	110mcg
azelastine	Astelin, Astepro	Nasal spray	IN	Allergies, anti-inflammatory	b.i.d.	137mcg, 205.5mcg
budesonide	Rhinocort	Nasal spray	IN	Allergies, anti-inflammatory	q.d.–b.i.d.	32mcg
chlorhexidine gluconate	Peridex, PerioGard	Liquid	Mouth	Antibacterial dental rinse	b.i.d.	0.12%
Nystatin	Nystatin	Liquid	PO	Antifungal	q.i.d.	10,000U/ml
fluoride	PreviDent 5000 Plus, EtheDent	Toothpaste	Teeth	Cavity protection	q.d.	1.1%
docosanol (OTC)	Abreva	Cream	Topical	Cold sores	5 times daily	10%
ciprofloxacin and dexamethasone	Ciprodex	Eardrop	Ear	Ear infection	b.i.d.	0.3%/0.1%
ciprofloxacin and hydrocortisone	Cipro HC otic	Eardrop	Ear	Ear infection	b.i.d.	0.2%/0.1%
ofloxacin	Floxin otic	Eardrop	Ear	Ear infection	q.d.	0.3%
oxymetazoline (OTC)	Afrin, Vicks Sinex, Sudafed OM	Nasal spray	IN	Nasal congestion	b.i.d.	0.05%
sodium chloride (OTC)	Ocean, Ayr	Nasal spray, gel	IN	Nasal congestion	PRN	0.5%
benzocaine (OTC)	Orajel, Benzodent, Anbesol, Orabase	Cream, gel	Mouth	Temporary pain relief	q.i.d.	7.5%, 10%, 20%
cyclosporine	Restasis	Eyedrop	Eye	To increase tear production	b.i.d.	0.05%
carbamide peroxide (OTC)	Debrox, Auro, Murine	Eardrop	Ear	To soften earwax	b.i.d.	6.5%
azelastine	Optivar	Eyedrop	Eye	To treat allergy symptoms	b.i.d.	0.05%
ketotifen fumarate	Zaditor	Eyedrop	Eye	To treat allergy symptoms	q.8–12h	0.025%
lodoxamide	Alomide	Eyedrop	Eye	To treat allergy symptoms	q.i.d.	0.1%
naphazoline (OTC)	Naphcon-A, Visine-A, Opcon-A	Eyedrop	Eye	To treat allergy symptoms	q.i.d.	0.025%

(Continued)

Table 12-1. Common Eyes, Ears, Nose, and Throat Agents and Their Uses (Continued)

Generic Name	Brand Name	Dosage Form	Route	Common Use	Common Frequency	Common Strengths
olopatadine	Pataday, Patanol	Eyedrop	Eye	To treat allergy symptoms	q.d., b.i.d.	0.1%, 0.2%
acetic acid	VoSoL	Eardrop	Ear	To treat ear infections	t.i.d.–q.i.d.	2%
acetic acid, propylene glycol diacetate, hydrocortisone	VoSoL HC	Eardrop	Ear	To treat ear infections	q.4–6h	2%/3%/1%
neomycin, polymyxin B, hydrocortisone	Cortisporin Otic	Eardrop	Ear	To treat ear infections	t.i.d.–q.i.d.	3.5mg/ 10,000U/10mg
bacitracin, neomycin, polymyxin B, hydrocortisone	Cortisporin	Ointment	Eye	To treat eye infections	q.3–4h	400U/3.5mg/ 10,000U/10mg
betaxolol	Betoptic S	Eyedrop	Eye	To treat glaucoma	b.i.d.	0.25%, 0.5%
bimatoprost	Lumigan	Eyedrop	Eye	To treat glaucoma	q.d.	0.03%
brimonidine	Alphagan P	Eyedrop	Eye	To treat glaucoma	q.8h	0.1%, 0.15%
brinzolamide	Azopt	Eyedrop	Eye	To treat glaucoma	t.i.d.	1%
dorzolamide	Trusopt	Eyedrop	Eye	To treat glaucoma	t.i.d.	2%
dorzolamide and timolol	Cosopt	Eyedrop	Eye	To treat glaucoma	b.i.d.	2%/0.5%
latanoprost	Xalatan	Eyedrop	Eye	To treat glaucoma	q.d.	0.005%
pilocarpine	Isopto Carpine, Pilocar	Eyedrop, gel	Eye	To treat glaucoma	1–6 times daily	0.5%, 1%, 2%, 4%
timolol	Timoptic	Eyedrop	Eye	To treat glaucoma	q.d., b.i.d.	0.25%, 0.5%
travoprost	Travatan, Travatan Z	Eyedrop	Eye	To treat glaucoma	q.d.	0.004%
ciprofloxacin	Ciloxan	Eyedrop, ointment	Eye	To treat ocular infections	q.2–4h, t.i.d.	0.3%
erythromycin	Erythromycin	Ointment	Eye	To treat ocular infections	2–6 times daily	0.5%
gatifloxacin	Zymar	Eyedrop	Eye	To treat ocular infections	q.2h–q.i.d.	0.3%
gentamicin	Gentak	Eyedrop, ointment	Eye	To treat ocular infections	q.2–4h, b.i.d., t.i.d.	0.3%
moxifloxacin	Vigamox	Eyedrop	Eye	To treat ocular infections	t.i.d.	0.5%
neomycin, polymyxin B, dexamethasone	Maxitrol	Eyedrop, ointment	Eye	To treat ocular infections	q.3–4h, t.i.d., q.i.d.	3.5mg/ 10,000U/0.1%
neomycin, polymyxin B, gramicidin	Neosporin	Eyedrop	Eye	To treat ocular infections	4–6 times daily	1.75mg/10,000U/ 0.025mg

(Continued)

Table 12-1. Common Eyes, Ears, Nose, and Throat Agents and Their Uses *(Continued)*

Generic Name	Brand Name	Dosage Form	Route	Common Use	Common Frequency	Common Strengths
sulfacetamide	Bleph-10	Eyedrop	Eye	To treat ocular infections	q.2–3h	10%
tobramycin	Tobrex	Eyedrop, ointment	Eye	To treat ocular infections	q.3–4h, b.i.d.–q.i.d.	0.3%
tobramycin and dexamethasone	TobraDex	Eyedrop, ointment	Eye	To treat ocular infections	q.2–6h, b.i.d.–q.i.d.	0.3%/0.1%
trimethoprim, polymyxin B	Polytrim	Eyedrop	Eye	To treat ocular infections	q.4–6h	1mg/10,000U
diclofenac	Voltaren Ophthalmic	Eyedrop	Eye	To treat ocular inflammation	q.i.d.	0.1%
fluorometholone	FML	Eyedrop	Eye	To treat ocular inflammation	b.i.d.–q.i.d.	0.1%
ketorolac	Acular	Eyedrop	Eye	To treat ocular inflammation	q.i.d.	0.4%, 0.5%
loteprednol	Lotemax	Eyedrop	Eye	To treat ocular inflammation	q.i.d.	0.2%/0.5%
prednisolone	Pred Forte, Pred Mild	Eyedrop	Eye	To treat ocular inflammation	b.i.d.–q.i.d.	0.12%, 1%
benzocaine and menthol (OTC)	Cepacol	Lozenge	Throat	To treat sore throat symptoms	q.2–4h PRN	10%/2mg
phenol (OTC)	Chloraseptic	Spray	Throat	To treat sore throat symptoms	q.2h PRN	1.4%

Dosage Forms, Routes of Administration, and Usual Doses for Eyes, Ears, Nose, Mouth, and Throat Medications

Many conditions affecting the eyes, ears, nose, mouth, and throat are treated locally, or at the site where the issue may occur. For instance, eyedrops are used to treat eye infections, eardrops are used to treat ear infections, and nasal sprays are used to alleviate nasal allergy symptoms. Direct application to the site may help to reduce overall side effects, because the medication does not have to travel through the whole body to reach the site of action.

Although creams and ointments are generally used on the skin, there are a few exceptions. Ointments can be used on the eye; an example of such an agent is ciprofloxacin eye ointment, which is used to treat infections. Creams, such as docosanol, can be applied to the mouth to treat cold sores.

To get medication to the throat, several dosage forms can be used. Nystatin can be given in liquid form and can be taken orally to coat the mouth and throat. Benzocaine and menthol come in lozenge form, which allows the medication to dissolve slowly in the mouth, providing a more constant release to the throat. Additionally, phenol in spray form can be used to coat the back of the throat directly, with minimal effect in the mouth.

Nasal medication applied directly to the nose may be the only effective route of administration for some agents. For instance, if sodium chloride is taken orally, it has far different effects than if it is applied directly to the nose. Some oral medications, such as Nystatin, work topically on infections of the mouth. Fluoride toothpastes and other oral products allow fluoride to be applied directly to the teeth where it is needed.

Common Side Effects of Eye, Ear, Nose, Mouth, and Throat Medications

Drops placed into the eye or ear are often used to get the medication directly to the site of infection or condition. Occasionally, blurred vision, itching, burning, and stinging may be noticed. Interestingly, taste issues may be also be noticed. Burning or stinging may be noticed when drops are placed in the eye, but this pain or irritation does not last long.

Terminology and Common Abbreviations Used with Eyes, Ears, Nose, Mouth, and Throat Medications

See Table 2-1, page 13, for abbreviations.

What's in a Name?

Table 12-2.	Examples of USAN Stems for Eye, Ear, Nose, Mouth, and Throat Medications	
Stem	**Description**	**Example**
-onide	Topical steroids (acetal derivatives)	ciclesonide
-cort-	Cortisone derivatives	hydrocortisone
-astine	Antihistaminics (histamine-H1 receptor antagonists)	azelastine
-zolamide	Carbonic anhydrase inhibitors	brinzolamide
-olol	Beta-blockers (propranolol type)	timolol

Technician Tip

Many eyedrop containers come in one or more fixed sizes. It is important to calculate the quantity necessary to fill the prescription to determine which size container should be dispensed, as well as the days supply based on the prescriber's directions. ℞

Sample Prescription for Eye, Ear, Nose, Mouth, and Throat Medications

DEA # BD0000000

John Doe, M.D.
123 Any Street
Any Town, Any State 00000
Tel. (123) 456-7890   Fax. (123) 456-1234

NAME _Kevin McGhee_

ADDRESS _1332 Saddlebrook_

℞   Vigamox #1 bottle

Sig: 1 drop OD TID x7d

_____J. Doe,_____ M.D.
(Signature)

REFILL _NR_

This prescription should be interpreted as Vigamox (moxifloxacin). Instill one drop in the right eye three times daily for seven days. Dispense 1 vial of solution (3ml) with no refills.

Technician Tip

It may be appropriate for a patient to not wear contact lenses during treatment with eyedrops. Also, some eyedrops must be refrigerated. Pharmacists may prefer to reinforce these points with auxiliary labels or patient counseling. If you are unsure if an auxiliary label is appropriate, ask your pharmacist. ℞

Alternative Therapies for Eye, Ear, Nose, Mouth, and Throat Conditions

Few alternative therapies exist for conditions affecting the eye, particularly to fight infection. However, there are several alternative options when treating conditions affecting ears. Some people who are susceptible to ear conditions such as swimmer's ear may use earplugs to prevent water from entering the ear. Also, some people who have recurrent earwax issues may need to clean their ears more frequently.

Oral infections are most often best left to standard prescription treatments. Several over-the-counter options exist for dental conditions to treat pain and prevent cavities; however, it is always important for patients to keep their dentist informed of any self-treatment strategies. Additionally, many home remedies exist for nasal congestion and common colds. Some may find Breathe Right strips useful to open up the nose externally and allow for air movement when suffering from nasal congestion. The SinuCleanse system and neti pots may also help to relieve sinus symptoms.

Chapter Summary !

Several dosage forms are available to treat various conditions of the eyes, ears, nose, mouth, and throat, generally by applying the drug directly to the site with the condition. Some examples include the following.

℞ Nasal sprays are available if nasal allergies are particularly problematic. These may be beneficial alternatives to oral medications, because side effects may be minimal while targeting the major symptoms

℞ Eyedrops can be used to treat glaucoma and eye infections, and eardrops can be used to treat ear infections

℞ Lozenges and sprays can be targeted at the throat to relieve pain associated with a sore throat

Additional nondrug therapies may be recommended to complement the direct application of medication to the affected site.

STUDENT NAME _____

DATE _____ INSTRUCTOR'S NAME _____

ANATOMY, PHYSIOLOGY, AND PHARMACOLOGY QUESTIONS:

Match the term to the site of use (circle one).

1. Otic   Eye   Ear

2. Ophthalmic   Eye   Ear

3. Ocular   Eye   Ear

Identify whether the following questions are true or false (circle one).

1. Ointments should never come into contact with the eye.

   TRUE   FALSE

2. Although medications may work in the same way if applied to different areas, dosages must be adjusted for the site.

   TRUE   FALSE

3. Direct application to the site may help to reduce side effects in other parts of the body.

   TRUE   FALSE

MEDICATION QUESTIONS

Match the following brand-name products with their generic names.

1. _____ Afrin
2. _____ Neosporin
3. _____ Maxitrol
4. _____ Acular
5. _____ Debrox
6. _____ Floxin Otic
7. _____ FML
8. _____ Xalatan

A. fluorometholone
B. ketorolac
C. latanoprost
D. neomycin, polymyxin B, and gramicidin
E. neomycin, polymyxin B, and dexamethasone
F. oxymetazoline
G. ofloxacin
H. carbamide peroxide

9. _____ NasalCrom
10. _____ Azopt
11. _____ Pred Forte
12. _____ Zaditor
13. _____ Vigamox
14. _____ Cosopt
15. _____ Optivar
16. _____ Tobrex

A. azelastine
B. cromolyn
C. brinzolamide
D. tobramycin
E. ketotifen fumarate
F. dorzolamide and timolol
G. prednisolone
H. moxifloxacin

17. _____ Ciloxan

18. _____ Abreva

19. _____ Orajel

20. _____ Nasacort

21. _____ Pilocar

22. _____ Polytrim

23. _____ PreviDent 5000 Plus

24. _____ Voltaren ophthalmic

A. pilocarpine

B. trimethoprim and polymyxin B

C. benzocaine

D. ciprofloxacin

E. fluoride

F. diclofenac

G. docosanol

H. triamcinolone

25. _____ Rhinocort

26. _____ Cortisporin

27. _____ Zymar

28. _____ Ciprodex

29. _____ Cortisporin Otic

30. _____ Ocean

31. _____ Lumigan

32. _____ VoSoL

A. gatifloxacin

B. sodium chloride

C. bimatoprost

D. ciprofloxacin and dexamethasone

E. acetic acid

F. budesonide

G. neomycin, polymyxin B, and hydrocortisone

H. bacitracin, neomycin, polymyxin B, and hydrocortisone

33. _____ VoSoL HC

34. _____ Travatan Z

35. _____ Trusopt

36. _____ Gentak

37. _____ Timoptic

38. _____ Pataday

39. _____ Betoptic S

40. _____ Alomide

A. timolol

B. acetic acid, propylene glycol diacetate, and hydrocortisone

C. travoprost

D. olopatadine

E. betaxolol

F. lodoxamide

G. dorzolamide

H. gentamicin

STUDENT NAME _____

DATE _____   INSTRUCTOR'S NAME _____

41. _____ Visine-A

42. _____ Peridex

43. _____ Alphagan P

44. _____ Restasis

45. _____ Bleph-10

46. _____ TobraDex

47. _____ Beconase

48. _____ Flonase

A. cyclosporine

B. naphazoline

C. beclomethasone

D. sulfacetamide

E. fluticasone

F. tobramycin and dexamethasone

G. chlorhexidine gluconate

H. brimonidine

49. _____ Cipro HC Otic

50. _____ Omnaris

51. _____ Cepacol

52. _____ Beconase

53. _____ Astelin

54. _____ Chloraseptic

55. _____ Lotemax

56. _____ Nasonex

A. phenol

B. benzocaine and menthol

C. ciprofloxacin and hydrocortisone

D. beclomethasone

E. ciclesonide

F. loteprednol

G. azelastine

H. mometasone

Select a common and appropriate frequency of administration (circle one).

1. diclofenac   q.d.   b.i.d.   t.i.d.   q.i.d.

2. Auro   q.d.   b.i.d.   t.i.d.   q.i.d.

3. Acular   q.d.   b.i.d.   t.i.d.   q.i.d.

4. dorzolamide   q.d.   b.i.d.   t.i.d.   q.i.d.

5. lodoxamide   q.d.   b.i.d.   t.i.d.   q.i.d.

6. Lumigan   q.d.   b.i.d.   t.i.d.   q.i.d.

7. PerioGard   q.d.   b.i.d.   t.i.d.   q.i.d.

8. Betoptic S   q.d.   b.i.d.   t.i.d.   q.i.d.

9. Floxin Otic   q.d.   b.i.d.   t.i.d.   q.i.d.

10. Vigamox   q.d.   b.i.d.   t.i.d.   q.i.d.

11. Afrin   q.d.   b.i.d.   t.i.d.   q.i.d.

12. Nasonex   q.d.   b.i.d.   t.i.d.   q.i.d.

Select the best available answer for the following questions.

1. Ciloxan is used to _____.

    a. treat inflammation
    b. treat glaucoma
    c. treat infection
    d. treat allergies

2. Opcon-A and Naphcon-A are both brand names for _____.

    a. phenol
    b. naphazoline
    c. cyclosporine
    d. ofloxacin

3. Veramyst is a drug that is used to _____.

    a. treat inflammation
    b. treat glaucoma
    c. treat infection
    d. treat allergies

4. Maxitrol is used to _____.

    a. treat inflammation
    b. treat glaucoma
    c. treat infection
    d. treat allergies

5. VoSoL HC contains _____.

    a. acetic acid, propylene glycol diacetate, and hydrocortisone
    b. neomycin, polymyxin B, and hydrocortisone
    c. bacitracin, neomycin, polymyxin B, and hydrocortisone
    d. ciprofloxacin and hydrocortisone

6. Ciprodex contains _____.

    a. ciprofloxacin and hydrocortisone
    b. trimethoprim and polymyxin B
    c. benzocaine and menthol
    d. ciprofloxacin and dexamethasone.

7. The generic name for Voltaren Ophthalmic is _____, and it is used to treat _____.

    a. olopatadine, ocular inflammation
    b. olopatadine, allergies
    c. diclofenac, ocular inflammation
    d. diclofenac, allergies

8. The proper site of administration of Cepacol is _____, and it is used to treat _____.

    a. throat, allergies
    b. nose, allergies
    c. throat, soreness
    d. nose, soreness

9. What do Rhinocort and Astelin have in common? _____

   a. Both are nasal sprays
   b. Both are tablets
   c. Both are eyedrops
   d. Both are eardrops

10. Anbesol and Benzodent both contain _____.

   a. benzocaine
   b. brinzolamide
   c. beclomethasone
   d. budesonide

11. Polytrim contains _____.

   a. tobramycin and dexamethasone
   b. neomycin, polymyxin B, and gramicidin
   c. trimethoprim and polymyxin B
   d. dorzolamide and timolol

12. The generic name of Chloraseptic is _____.

   a. sodium chloride
   b. oxymetazoline
   c. docosanol
   d. phenol

13. Gentak is used to _____.

   a. treat inflammation
   b. treat glaucoma
   c. treat infection
   d. treat allergies

14. Olopatadine is generic for _____.

   a. Pataday
   b. Pilocar
   c. Pred Mild
   d. Ayr

15. Pilocar is available as _____.

   a. an eyedrop
   b. an eardrop
   c. a toothpaste
   d. a spray

12. EXERCISES

DISCUSSION AND CRITICAL THINKING QUESTIONS:

1. What are some ways that allergies present?

2. What are some cases when ointments might not be used on the skin?

3. What are some products that could help with symptom relief from a cold but that are not medications taken orally?

4. Why is it sometimes better to apply antibiotics directly to the eye or ear, rather than taking an oral antibiotic?

5. Allergies may cause nasal symptoms. What are some lifestyle changes that one might try to reduce allergy symptoms?

STUDENT NAME _____

DATE _____ INSTRUCTOR'S NAME _____

SAMPLE PRESCRIPTIONS

DEA # BD0000000

John Doe, M.D.
123 Any Street
Any Town, Any State 00000
Tel. (123) 456-7890   Fax. (123) 456-1234

NAME   _Leonard Spengler_____

ADDRESS   _2383 Haverford_____

Rx   Xalatan #1 bottle

Sig: 1 drop OU QHS

_____ J. Doe,   M.D.
                        (Signature)

REFILL   _RFx1_____

NDC 0013-8303-04
Rx only
One 2.5 mL Bottle

Xalatan®
latanoprost ophthalmic solution

STERILE
0.005%

125 µg/2.5 mL*

Distributed by
Pfizer **Pharmacia & Upjohn Co**
Division of Pfizer Inc, NY, NY 10017

1. What is the generic name for Xalatan?

_____

_____

2. How would you translate the Sig code into plain English so that the patient could understand the directions for use?

_____

_____

_____

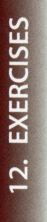

12. EXERCISES

3. How many refills are given on this prescription?

_____

_____

_____

4. If Xalatan comes in 2.5ml containers, and each milliliter provides 15 drops, how many drops are included per container?

_____

_____

_____

5. What is the days supply for this prescription? _____
   A: 30 days
   B: 25 days
   C: 18 days
   D: 10 days

STUDENT NAME _____

DATE _____ INSTRUCTOR'S NAME _____

DEA # BD0000000

John Doe, M.D.
123 Any Street
Any Town, Any State 00000
Tel. (123) 456-7890   Fax. (123) 456-1234

NAME   *Nate Clarkston* _____

ADDRESS   *1922 Fenway* _____

Rx   *Cipro HC Otic #1 bottle*

Sig: *3 drops a.s. b.i.d. x7d*

_____ *J. Doe,* _____ M.D.
(Signature)

REFILL   *NR* _____

1. What is the generic name for Cipro HC Otic?

   _____

   _____

2. How would you translate the Sig code into plain English so that the patient could understand the directions for use?

   _____

   _____

   _____

3. How many refills are given on this prescription?

_____

_____

_____

_____

4. What is a common use for this medication?

_____

_____

_____

_____

5. If a 10ml bottle was dispensed, and each milliliter provides 15 drops, how many drops are contained in each bottle?

_____

_____

_____

_____

6. If the physician wanted the patient to continue using the medication past the original directions, how many days could this product last?

_____

_____

_____

_____

STUDENT NAME _____

DATE _____ INSTRUCTOR'S NAME _____

DEA # BD0000000

John Doe, M.D.
123 Any Street
Any Town, Any State 00000
Tel. (123) 456-7890   Fax. (123) 456-1234

NAME ___Frank Apollo_____

ADDRESS ___1442 Florida Ln._____

R̲x   Abreva #1 tube

Sig: A AA 5x daily

_____ J. Doe, _____ M.D.
                    (Signature)

REFILL ___NR_____

1. What is the generic name for Abreva?

   _____

   _____

2. How would you translate the Sig code into plain English so that the patient could understand the directions for use?

   _____

   _____

   _____

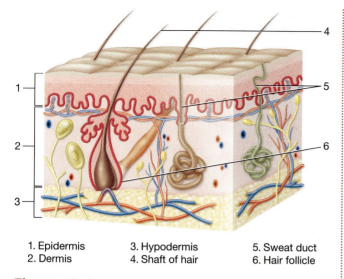

1. Epidermis   3. Hypodermis   5. Sweat duct
2. Dermis   4. Shaft of hair   6. Hair follicle

Figure 13-1. Skin section.

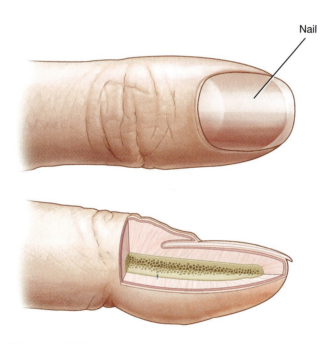

Nail

Figure 13-2. Nail anatomy.

Parts of the skin section shown include epidermis, dermis, hypodermis, shaft of hair, sweat duct, and hair follicle. Figure 13-2 shows nail anatomy.

Parts of the hair structure shown in Figure 13-1 include: shaft of hair, sweat duct, and hair follicle.

Knowing the following terms will be helpful as you learn about the medications used to treat conditions affecting the dermatologic system.

Acne: a skin condition characterized by scaly red skin, blackheads and whiteheads, pimples, and sometimes inflammation

Athlete's foot: a common fungal infection of the skin

Dermatologic: Pertaining to the skin and its structure, functions, and diseases

Impetigo: a contagious bacterial infection of the skin

Integumentary system: system containing the skin, hair, and nails

Jock itch: a common fungal infection of the skin

Keratoses: crusty or scaly patches of skin

Ringworm: a common fungal infection of the skin

Sulfa drug: a type of antibiotic

Primer on Pharmacologic Actions of Dermatologic Agents

Dermatologic agents are medications used to treat conditions of the skin, hair, and nails. They treat a range of conditions, including infections, itching, acne, keratoses, rashes, burns, diaper rash, sun exposure, and facial wrinkling.

The most common infections of the skin are bacterial and fungal infections. Impetigo is one type of contagious bacterial infection of the skin and can be treated topically with mupirocin (Bactroban). There are other types of bacterial infections of the skin, and their treatment depends on the type of infection that is present. Athlete's foot, jock itch, and ringworm are common contagious fungal infections of the skin. Ketoconazole (Nizoral) is an antifungal drug used to treat fungal infections of the skin.

Acne is a skin condition characterized by scaly red skin, blackheads and whiteheads, pimples, and sometimes inflammation. Different treatments for acne work in different ways. Benzoyl peroxide (Benzac, Desquam, and others) is one example of a medication that is commonly used to treat acne.

Keratoses are crusty or scaly patches of skin. Fluorouracil (Efudex) is an example of a medication used to treat keratoses.

Rashes can have a variety of causes, including poison ivy, poison oak, insect bites, soaps, and detergents. Hydrocortisone (Cortaid) is a topical corticosteroid that can help with the symptoms of a rash.

Burns to the skin vary in their severity. Burns that extend into deeper layers of the skin require treatment to prevent bacterial infections. Silver sulfadiazine

(Silvadene) is a sulfa drug that is applied to the skin to treat infections of second- and third-degree burns.

Zinc oxide is an important ingredient in baby powders, as well as in ointments and creams used to treat diaper rash. In creams and ointments, zinc oxide functions as a barrier to protect the skin. Sun expo-

sure can also be blocked by zinc oxide in ointments and creams.

Facial wrinkling that can be associated with aging can be treated by tretinoin (Retin-A). Tretinoin is more commonly used to treat acne, but it can also repair damage to the skin caused by sunlight.

Table 13-1. Common Dermatologic Agents and Their Uses

Generic Name	Brand Name	Dosage Form	Route	Common Use	Common Frequency	Common Strengths
silver sulfadiazine	Silvadene	Cream	Topical	A sulfa drug used to prevent and treat infections of second- and third-degree burns	q.d.–b.i.d.	1%
clobetasol propionate	Temovate	Cream, ointment	Topical	For the temporary relief of minor skin irritations, itching, and rashes	b.i.d.	0.05%
desoximetasone	Topicort	Cream	Topical	For the temporary relief of minor skin irritations, itching, and rashes	b.i.d.	0.25%
fluocinolone	Synalar	Cream	Topical	For the temporary relief of minor skin irritations, itching, and rashes	b.i.d.–q.i.d.	0.025%
fluocinonide	Lidex	Cream, ointment	Topical	For the temporary relief of minor skin irritations, itching, and rashes	b.i.d.–q.i.d.	0.2%
fluticasone propionate	Cutivate	Cream, ointment	Topical	For the temporary relief of minor skin irritations, itching, and rashes	q.d.–b.i.d.	0.005%, 0.05%
hydrocortisone (OTC)	Cortaid	Cream	Topical	For the temporary relief of minor skin irritations, itching, and rashes	b.i.d.–t.i.d.	0.5%, 1%, 2.5%
hydrocortisone valerate	Westcort	Cream, ointment	Topical	For the temporary relief of minor skin irritations, itching, and rashes	b.i.d.–t.i.d.	0.2%
mometasone furoate	Elocon	Cream, ointment	Topical	For the temporary relief of minor skin irritations, itching, and rashes	q.d.	0.1%
triamcinolone	Kenalog	Cream, ointment	Topical	For the temporary relief of minor skin irritations, itching, and rashes	t.i.d.–q.i.d.	0.025%, 0.1%, 0.5%
diphenhydramine	Benadryl	Cream, gel	Topical	To block the actions of histamines	t.i.d.–q.i.d.	1%, 2%
bacitracin (OTC)	Baciguent	Ointment	Topical	To prevent minor skin injuries from becoming infected	q.d.–q.i.d.	500U/g
neomycin, polymyxin, and bacitracin (OTC)	Neosporin	Ointment	Topical	To prevent minor skin injuries from becoming infected	q.d.–t.i.d.	3.5mg/ 5000U/400U
zinc oxide (OTC)	Desitin	Cream	Topical	To protect and heal diaper rash	PRN	40%
zinc oxide (OTC)	Zinc oxide	Cream, spray	Topical	To protect the skin from sun exposure	PRN	Based on SPF scale
Adapalene	Differin	Cream, solution, gel	Topical	To treat acne	q.d.	0.1%
Clindamycin	Cleocin	Gel, lotion	Topical	To treat acne	b.i.d.	1%
clindamycin and benzoyl peroxide	BenzaClin, Duac	Gel	Topical	To treat acne	b.i.d.	1%/5%

(Continued)

Technician Tip

Benzoyl peroxide/erythromycin must be reconstituted and is only good for three months after reconstitution. Additionally, it must be refrigerated after reconstitution. Your pharmacist may not want this medication to be reconstituted until the patient arrives to pick up the medication. Check with your pharmacist if you are unsure whether you should reconstitute benzoyl peroxide/erythromycin. ℞

Alternative Therapies for Dermatologic Conditions

Many home remedies and alternative therapies exist for the treatment of acne, including the use of cleansers and the avoidance of triggers, such as certain foods. The treatment of lice requires alternative action, including the washing of bedding and clothing that may harbor lice during the patient's treatment. Although infections often require treatment with a medication, alternative therapies may also be appropriate in conjunction with the medical treatment. For instance, it may be helpful for someone with athlete's foot to change his or her socks regularly and to alternate pairs of shoes every other day.

Chapter Summary !

Dermatologic conditions are often treated with topical therapies, although oral medications can also be used. Some examples of dermatologic treatments include the following.

℞ Several prescription and over-the-counter acne treatments are available. They are often applied topically, but isotretinoin can also be used as an oral agent. If isotretinoin is used, the patient must be registered with the *iPLEDGE* program

℞ Dandruff and lice may be treated with shampoos to apply the medication directly to the site

℞ Topical treatments for skin infections include antifungals for conditions such as athlete's foot, jock itch, and ringworm. Antibacterial products may be used for impetigo

Self-treatment is common with dermatologic agents, so patients may come to the pharmacy counter with questions about the most appropriate uses for agents. Pharmacists may counsel many patients for self-care of such dermatologic conditions.

STUDENT NAME _____

DATE _____ INSTRUCTOR'S NAME _____

ANATOMY, PHYSIOLOGY, AND PHARMACOLOGY QUESTIONS

Identify whether the following are bacterial or fungal infections (circle one).

1. Athlete's foot   Bacterial   Fungal
2. Ringworm   Bacterial   Fungal
3. Impetigo   Bacterial   Fungal
4. Jock itch   Bacterial   Fungal

Identify if the following questions are true or false (circle one).

1. Zinc oxide may serve several purposes, including protection from the sun and treatment of diaper rash.
    TRUE   FALSE

2. Topical corticosteroids may help treat rash symptoms.
    TRUE   FALSE

3. Some more severe burns may require treatment to prevent bacterial infection.
    TRUE   FALSE

MEDICATION QUESTIONS:

Match the following brand-name products with their generic names.

1. _____ Synalar
2. _____ Duac
3. _____ Efudex
4. _____ Differin
5. _____ Tazorac
6. _____ Rid
7. _____ Lamisil
8. _____ Westcort

A. clindamycin and benzoyl peroxide
B. permethrin
C. terbinafine
D. adapalene
E. fluorouracil
F. fluocinolone
G. hydrocortisone valerate
H. tazarotene

9. _____ Lidex
10. _____ Topicort
11. _____ Aldara
12. _____ OXY
13. _____ Selsun Blue
14. _____ Bactroban
15. _____ Neosporin
16. _____ Lotrisone

A. fluocinonide
B. imiquimod
C. desoximetasone
D. mupirocin
E. selenium disulfide
F. neomycin, polymyxin, and bacitracin
G. benzoyl peroxide
H. betamethasone dipropionate, clotrimazole

17. _____ Cortaid
18. _____ Cutivate
19. _____ Triaz
20. _____ Elocon
21. _____ Cleocin
22. _____ Silvadene
23. _____ Kenalog
24. _____ Amnesteem

A. benzoyl peroxide
B. isotretinoin
C. clindamycin
D. fluticasone propionate
E. silver sulfadiazine
F. triamcinolone
G. hydrocortisone
H. mometasone furoate

25. _____ Zovirax
26. _____ Benadryl
27. _____ Temovate
28. _____ Claravis
29. _____ Baciguent
30. _____ Nizoral
31. _____ Benoxyl
32. _____ Head and Shoulders

A. clobetasol propionate
B. benzoyl peroxide
C. isotretinoin
D. pyrithione zinc
E. bacitracin
F. acyclovir
G. ketoconazole
H. diphenhydramine

33. _____ Benzamycin
34. _____ Retin-A
35. _____ Benzac
36. _____ Sotret
37. _____ Desitin
38. _____ Medrol

A. isotretinoin
B. benzoyl peroxide
C. zinc oxide
D. tretinoin
E. methylprednisolone
F. erythromycin and benzoyl peroxide

STUDENT NAME _____

DATE _____ INSTRUCTOR'S NAME _____

Select a common and appropriate frequency of administration (circle one).

1. terbinafine	q.d.	b.i.d.	t.i.d.	PRN
2. BenzaClin	q.d.	b.i.d.	t.i.d.	PRN
3. zinc oxide	q.d.	b.i.d.	t.i.d.	PRN
4. Bactroban	q.d.	b.i.d.	t.i.d.	PRN
5. Elocon	q.d.	b.i.d.	t.i.d.	PRN
6. Lotrisone	q.d.	b.i.d.	t.i.d.	PRN
7. tretinoin	q.d.	b.i.d.	t.i.d.	PRN
8. isotretinoin	q.d.	b.i.d.	t.i.d.	PRN
9. Topicort	q.d.	b.i.d.	t.i.d.	PRN
10. adapalene	q.d.	b.i.d.	t.i.d.	PRN

Select the appropriate main use/drug class (circle one).

1. Nix	Acne	Fungal infections	Lice
2. ketoconazole	Acne	Fungal infections	Lice
3. Benzamycin	Acne	Fungal infections	Lice
4. Neutrogena	Acne	Fungal infections	Lice
5. lindane	Acne	Fungal infections	Lice
6. Differin	Acne	Fungal infections	Lice
7. permethrin	Acne	Fungal infections	Lice
8. Lamisil	Acne	Fungal infections	Lice
9. isotretinoin	Acne	Fungal infections	Lice
10. clindamycin	Acne	Fungal infections	Lice
11. mometasone furoate	Skin irritations	Acne	
12. Desquam	Skin irritations	Acne	
13. fluocinolone	Skin irritations	Acne	
14. Kenalog	Skin irritations	Acne	
15. Tazorac	Skin irritations	Acne	
16. Cleocin	Skin irritations	Acne	
17. BenzaClin	Skin irritations	Acne	
18. Lidex	Skin irritations	Acne	
19. clobetasol propionate	Skin irritations	Acne	
20. ZoDerm	Skin irritations	Acne	

Identify whether the following questions are true or false (circle one).

1. Claravis is applied topically to treat acne.

   TRUE   FALSE

2. Fluticasone propionate is used for minor skin irritations.

   TRUE   FALSE

3. Aldara cream is used to treat warts.

   TRUE   FALSE

4. Retin-A can be used to treat wrinkles.

   TRUE   FALSE

5. Acyclovir is used topically to treat cold sores.

   TRUE   FALSE

6. Silvadene is used to treat dandruff.

   TRUE   FALSE

7. Efudex is dosed b.i.d.

   TRUE   FALSE

8. Medrol is used to treat inflammation.

   TRUE   FALSE

9. Pyrithione zinc and selenium disulfide are both used PRN to treat a sunburn.

   TRUE   FALSE

10. Bacitracin is used to prevent infections following minor skin injuries.

    TRUE   FALSE

Select the best available answer for the following questions.

1. Zinc oxide is often used topically to _____.
   a. protect from the sun
   b. treat acne
   c. treat dandruff
   d. treat warts

2. Zovirax is commonly dosed _____.
   a. 1–2 times daily
   b. 3–4 times daily
   c. 5–6 times daily
   d. 7–8 times daily

3. Lindane is given _____.

    a. intravenously

    b. orally

    c. topically

    d. intramuscularly

4. Neosporin is used to _____ skin infections and is given _____.

    a. treat, orally

    b. prevent, orally

    c. prevent, topically

    d. treat, topically

5. Westcort and Elocon can both be used to treat _____.

    a. acne

    b. fungal infections

    c. facial wrinkles

    d. minor skin irritations

6. Imiquimod is dosed _____ and can be used to treat _____.

    a. Once weekly, acne

    b. Twice weekly, warts

    c. Twice daily, acne

    d. Minor skin irritations

7. Clobetasol propionate is dosed _____.

    a. q.d.

    b. b.i.d.

    c. t.i.d.

    d. q.i.d.

8. Selenium disulfide is given _____.

    a. b.i.d.

    b. q.d.

    c. q.week

    d. PRN

9. Which of the following can be used to treat wrinkles? _____

    a. diphenhydramine

    b. benzoyl peroxide

    c. isotretinoin

    d. tretinoin

10. Triaz, ZoDerm, NeoBenz, and Benoxyl all contain _____.

    a. benzoyl peroxide

    b. diphenhydramine

    c. bacitracin

    d. fluticasone

13. EXERCISES

DISCUSSION AND CRITICAL THINKING QUESTIONS

1. What brand names of acne products are sold in your pharmacy? What are their active ingredients?

2. Which topical products might your pharmacy stock extra and advertise in the summer?

3. Not all topical products may be sold near the pharmacy. Where are some other areas of the store where topical products may be sold?

4. Why do non-childbearing-age females and males need to participate in the iPLEDGE program?

5. What training does your pharmacy require regarding the iPLEDGE system?

STUDENT NAME _____

DATE _____ INSTRUCTOR'S NAME _____

3. Lindane is given _____.
   a. intravenously
   b. orally
   c. topically
   d. intramuscularly

4. Neosporin is used to _____ skin infections and is given _____.
   a. treat, orally
   b. prevent, orally
   c. prevent, topically
   d. treat, topically

5. Westcort and Elocon can both be used to treat _____.
   a. acne
   b. fungal infections
   c. facial wrinkles
   d. minor skin irritations

6. Imiquimod is dosed _____ and can be used to treat _____.
   a. Once weekly, acne
   b. Twice weekly, warts
   c. Twice daily, acne
   d. Minor skin irritations

7. Clobetasol propionate is dosed _____.
   a. q.d.
   b. b.i.d.
   c. t.i.d.
   d. q.i.d.

8. Selenium disulfide is given _____.
   a. b.i.d.
   b. q.d.
   c. q.week
   d. PRN

9. Which of the following can be used to treat wrinkles? _____
   a. diphenhydramine
   b. benzoyl peroxide
   c. isotretinoin
   d. tretinoin

10. Triaz, ZoDerm, NeoBenz, and Benoxyl all contain _____.
    a. benzoyl peroxide
    b. diphenhydramine
    c. bacitracin
    d. fluticasone

13. EXERCISES

DISCUSSION AND CRITICAL THINKING QUESTIONS

1. What brand names of acne products are sold in your pharmacy? What are their active ingredients?

2. Which topical products might your pharmacy stock extra and advertise in the summer?

3. Not all topical products may be sold near the pharmacy. Where are some other areas of the store where topical products may be sold?

4. Why do non-childbearing-age females and males need to participate in the iPLEDGE program?

5. What training does your pharmacy require regarding the iPLEDGE system?

STUDENT NAME _____

DATE _____ INSTRUCTOR'S NAME _____

SAMPLE PRESCRIPTIONS:

DEA # BD0000000

John Doe, M.D.
123 Any Street
Any Town, Any State 00000
Tel. (123) 456-7890   Fax. (123) 456-1234

NAME _____Dan Hill_____

ADDRESS ___148 Snail Dr._____

℞   Silvadene 1% #50g

Sig: A AA BID

_____J. Doe,_____ M.D.
(Signature)

REFILL ___NR_____

---

1. What is the generic name for Silvadene?

   _____

   _____

2. How would you translate the Sig code into plain English so that the patient could understand the directions for use?

   _____

   _____

   _____

3. How many refills are given on this prescription?

_____

_____

_____

_____

4. What amount of drug should be dispensed?

_____

_____

_____

_____

5. What common condition(s) does this medication treat?

_____

_____

_____

_____

STUDENT NAME _____

DATE _____ INSTRUCTOR'S NAME _____

DEA # BD0000000

John Doe, M.D.
123 Any Street
Any Town, Any State 00000
Tel. (123) 456-7890   Fax. (123) 456-1234

NAME _Mike Wilson_____

ADDRESS _2284 Northcoast Ln._____

Rx   Medrol Dosepak 4mg #21

Sig: UTD

_____ J. Doe, _____ M.D.
                    (Signature)

REFILL _NR_____

NDC 0009-0056-04

21 Tablets   Rx only

Medrol® Dosepak™
methylprednisolone
tablets, USP

4 mg
Unit of Use

Pfizer Distributed by
Pharmacia & Upjohn Co
Division of Pfizer Inc, NY, NY 10017

---

1. What is the generic name for Medrol?

   _____

   _____

2. How would you translate the Sig code into plain English so that the patient could understand the directions for use?

   _____

   _____

3. How many refills are given on this prescription?

4. What other common strengths are available for Medrol oral tablets?

5. What is a common use for this medication?

STUDENT NAME _____

DATE _____ INSTRUCTOR'S NAME _____

DEA # BD0000000

John Doe, M.D.
123 Any Street
Any Town, Any State 00000
Tel. (123) 456-7890   Fax. (123) 456-1234

NAME _Katherine McVick_____

ADDRESS _2127 Pike Ct._____

Rx   Zovirax Cream #2g

Sig: A cold sores 5x daily x4d

_____ J. Doe, _____ M.D.
(Signature)

REFILL _Rfx 1_____

1. What is the generic name for Zovirax?

   _____

   _____

2. How would you translate the Sig code into plain English so that the patient could understand the directions for use?

   _____

   _____

   _____

3. How many refills are given on this prescription?

4. What is a common use for this medication?

Hematology and Oncology Medications

14

KEY TERMS

Anemia

Aplastic anemia

Benign tumor

Chemotherapy

Clotting factor

Erythrocytes

Hematology

Hemophilia

Hemostatic agents

Leukocytes

Malignant tumor

Metastasis

Oncology

Plasma

Platelets

Thrombocytes

LEARNING OBJECTIVES

After completing this chapter, the student will be able to:

1. Describe the basic anatomy and physiology of the hematologic system

2. Explain the term *cancer*

3. Explain the therapeutic effects of common medications used to treat cancer and diseases of the hematologic system

4. List the brand and generic names of common medications used to treat cancer and diseases of the hematologic system

5. List the brand and generic names of common medications used to treat cancer and diseases of the hematologic system

6. Identify available dosage forms for common cancer and hematologic system medications

7. Identify routes of administration for common cancer and hematologic system medications

8. Identify usual doses for common cancer and hematologic system medications

9. List common side effects of frequently prescribed cancer and hematologic system medications

10. Define medical terms commonly used when treating cancer and diseases of the hematologic system

11. List abbreviations for terms associated with the use of medication therapy for cancer and common diseases affecting the hematologic system

12. Describe alternative therapies commonly used to treat cancer and diseases of the hematologic system

Basic Anatomy and Physiology of the Hematologic System

The blood has critical functions in the body. The study of blood, the blood-forming organs, and blood diseases is called *hematology*. Blood is a mixture of cells suspended in a liquid material called plasma. The plasma consists of water, nutrients, hormones, salts, proteins, and waste products. Besides plasma, there are three other main components of blood:

1. Red blood cells (RBCs, erythrocytes)
2. White blood cells (WBCs, leukocytes)
3. Platelets (thrombocytes)

Red blood cells are primarily responsible for delivering oxygen from the lungs to tissues and organs throughout the body. Red blood cells are made in the bone marrow, which is found inside the bones. See Figure 14-1 for a view of a long bone and the location of bone marrow.

White blood cells are part of the body's defense system and have an important role in fighting infections. Lymphocytes are formed in lymphatic tissue throughout the body, including the spleen, thymus, tonsils, and lymph nodes.

Platelets are important for blood clotting to occur. Platelets are also made in the bone marrow (Figure 14-1).

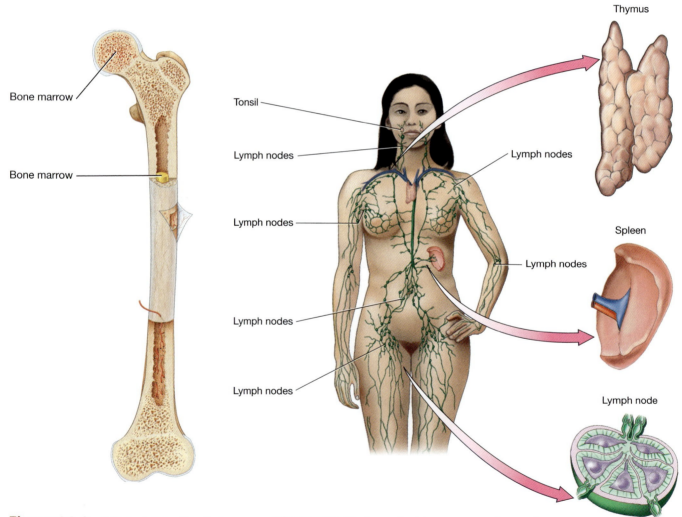

Figure 14-1. A long bone: the femur.

Figure 14-2. Lymphoid organs and vessels.

Blood Disorders

The most common blood disorders are bleeding disorders and anemia. The blood-clotting process involves platelets as well as proteins in the blood known as clotting factors. Bleeding disorders are due to deficiencies in platelets or clotting factors. Hemophilia is one type of bleeding disorder in which the blood does not clot normally because of a clotting factor deficiency. Anemia is a condition in which the blood does not carry enough oxygen to body tissues. The most common causes of anemia are not having enough iron, folic acid, or vitamin B_{12} in the diet. Cancer can also cause anemia. Symptoms of anemia are weakness, feeling cold, dizziness, and irritability. The type of anemia is confirmed by testing the blood, and treatment is determined by the type of anemia.

Cancer

A tumor is an abnormal new growth of tissue that possesses no physiological function. One important function of the immune system is to identify and eliminate tumors (see Chapter 4 for information about the anatomy and physiology of the immune system). Tumors can be characterized as benign or malignant. A benign tumor is a mild type of abnormal new growth of tissue with no physiologic function that does not threaten health. Malignant tumors are more serious than benign tumors; they usually threaten health and can lead to death. Malignant tumors are also known as cancer. The study of cancer is called oncology. Malignant tumors can break away and spread to other parts of the body. Metastasis is a term to describe when cancer spreads to one or more other parts of the body. How cancers are named is determined by where the cancerous growth starts. Chemotherapy is a term used to describe the treatment of cancer with medications.

Knowing the following terms will be helpful as you learn about the medications used to treat diseases of the hematologic system and cancer.

Anemia: Anemia is a condition in which the blood does not carry enough oxygen to body tissues

Aplastic anemia: A condition in which the bone marrow does not produce enough blood cells

Benign tumor: A mild type of abnormal new tissue growth that has no physiologic function that does not threaten health

Chemotherapy: A term used for the treatment of cancer with medications

Clotting factors: Proteins in the blood that work with platelets to produce blood clots

Erythrocytes: Red blood cells (RBCs)

Hematology: The study of blood, the blood-forming organs, and blood diseases

Hemophilia: One type of bleeding disorder in which the blood does not clot normally because of clotting factor deficiency

Hemostatic agents: Medications that slow some types of bleeding by slowing the rate of the breakdown of blood clots

Leukocytes: White blood cells (WBCs)

Malignant tumor: Abnormal new growth of tissue that has no physiologic function; malignant tumors usually threaten health and can lead to death

Metastasis: A term to describe the spread of cancer to one or more other parts of the body

Oncology: The study of cancer

Plasma: The liquid component of blood, which consists of water, nutrients, hormones, salts, proteins, and waste products

Platelets: A type of blood cell made in the bone marrow that plays an important role in blood clotting (also known as thrombocytes)

Thrombocytes: A type of blood cell made in the bone marrow that plays an important role in blood clotting (also known as platelets)

Primer on Pharmacologic Actions of Hematology and Oncology Agents

Hematology medications can generally be thought of as drugs that are used to treat bleeding disorders and anemias. Bleeding disorders include hemophilia and other problems associated with blood clotting.

Some bleeding disorders, certain types of cancer, and some surgeries involving the heart or liver can be accompanied by a condition in which blood clots are broken down too quickly. This results in excessive bleeding. Aminocaproic acid (Amicar) is a drug used to treat this condition. Aminocaproic acid and tranexamic acid (Cyklokapron) are examples of hemostatic agents that work by slowing the rate of the breakdown of blood clots.

Some blood clotting problems are associated with a deficiency of vitamin K in the body. Vitamin K is needed for blood to clot normally. Phytonadione (vitamin K) is used to prevent bleeding in people with vitamin K deficiency.

A variety of anemias can result in having an inadequate supply of oxygen throughout the body. The most common causes of anemias are not having enough iron, folic acid, or vitamin B_{12}. Iron is available in a number of forms, including ferrous sulfate, ferrous fumarate, iron polysaccharide, and ferrous gluconate. Iron is used by the body in the production of red blood cells. Iron-deficiency anemia can be caused by inadequate diet, pregnancy, excess bleeding, as well as other medical problems. Folic acid is also used in the body in the production of red blood cells, and a deficiency of this vitamin can lead to a deficiency in red blood cells. Vitamin B_{12} also plays a role in the production of red blood cells. Some people do not effectively absorb vitamin B_{12} in the diet and must be given vitamin B_{12} injections to maintain an adequate production of red blood cells. Chronic kidney failure and certain types of chemotherapy can result in red blood cell deficiency. Epoetin alfa (Epogen) is used to increase the production of red blood cells in the bone marrow. Additionally, epoetin alfa is sometimes used before and after certain types of surgery so that fewer blood transfusions are needed. Aplastic anemia is a form of anemia in which the bone marrow does not produce enough blood cells. Anti-thymocyte globulin (Thymoglobulin) is used in the treatment of aplastic anemia and in the prevention and treatment of acute rejection in organ transplantation. Cancer can also cause anemia by decreasing the number of certain types of white blood cells and increasing the chance of infection. Filgrastim (Neupogen) is a medication that helps the body make a certain type of white blood cells.

Although a few specific vitamins such as vitamin B_{12}, folic acid, and vitamin K have been described to have therapeutic benefits for some specific hematologic conditions, other vitamins, in the form of multivitamins, are also sometimes prescribed. Vitamins are naturally occurring substances that need to be ingested for normal growth, development, and functioning of the body. For most people, a well-balanced diet usually provides an adequate amount of vitamins. Centrum is an example of a multivitamin that is sometimes prescribed when vitamin supplementation is needed. Also, during pregnancy, the requirement for certain vitamins increases. Prenatal multivitamins such as Primacare One are formulated for the vitamin requirements typically associated with pregnancy.

Oncology medications can generally be thought of as chemotherapy agents. The treatment of cancer is often complex. The type of cancer along with how advanced it is are used to determine treatment plans. Treatment plans may include surgery, radiation, chemotherapy, or a combination of these. Chemotherapy agents are powerful drugs and often require special handling.

Some common hematology and oncology agents and their uses are listed in Table 14-1. Some common chemotherapy agents are listed in Table 14-2.

Technician Tip

Medications used to treat cancer are often used in combination with other agents. The suggested combinations change frequently, which may change the individual dose or schedule of the medication. It is important to monitor carefully the exact dose and schedule of an agent, as well as the medications it is paired with for a specific patient, because routine combinations may change frequently. ℞

Table 14-1. Common Hematology and Oncology Agents and Their Uses

Generic Name	Brand Name	Dosage Form	Route	Common Use	Common Frequency	Common Strengths
aminocaproic acid	Amicar	Tablet, liquid, parenteral	PO, IV	To control bleeding from blood clots that were broken down too quickly	q.4–6h	500mg, 1000mg, 250mg/ml
phytonadione (vitamin K₁)	Mephyton	Tablet, parenteral	PO, IV, IM, SQ	To prevent bleeding in people with blood clotting problems	q.d., PRN	100mg, 1mg/0.5ml, 10mg/ml
tranexamic acid	Cyklokapron	Tablet, parenteral	PO, IV	To prevent bleeding in people with hemophilia	t.i.d.	650mg, 100mg/ml
ferrous fumarate	Femiron, Ferretts	Tablet	PO	To treat or prevent iron-deficiency anemia	q.d.	63mg, 150mg, 200mg, 325mg
ferrous gluconate	Fergon	Tablet	PO	To treat or prevent iron-deficiency anemia	q.d.–q.i.d.	240mg, 246mg, 324mg, 325mg
ferrous sulfate	Feosol, Fer-In-Sol, Slow FE	Tablet, liquid	PO	To treat or prevent iron-deficiency anemia	q.d.–q.i.d.	160mg, 200mg, 325mg, 75mg/ml
iron polysaccharide	Niferex	Capsule, liquid	PO	To treat or prevent iron-deficiency anemia	q.d.–b.i.d.	60mg, 150mg, 180mg, 100mg/5ml
iron sucrose	Venofer	Parenteral	IV	To treat or prevent iron-deficiency anemia	1-3 times weekly, every other week	20mg/ml
cyanocobalamin	Vitamin B₁₂	Tablet, parenteral, nasal spray	PO, IN,	To treat or prevent vitamin B₁₂ deficiency	q.d., q.week, q.month	50mcg, 100mcg, 250mcg, 500mcg, 1000mcg, 2500mcg, 5000mcg, 1000mcg/ml
filgrastim	Neupogen	Parenteral	IV, SQ	Treatment of a low white blood cell count due to cancer	q.d.	300mcg, 480mcg
pegfilgrastim	Neulasta	Parenteral	SQ	Treatment of a low white blood cell count due to cancer	Once per chemotherapy cycle	6mg

(Continued)

Table 14-1. Common Hematology and Oncology Agents and Their Uses *(Continued)*

Generic Name	Brand Name	Dosage Form	Route	Common Use	Common Frequency	Common Strengths
darbepoetin Alfa	Aranesp	Parenteral	IV, SQ	Treatment of anemia due to kidney failure or cancer	q.week	25mcg, 40mcg, 60mcg, 100mcg, 150mcg
epoetin alfa	Epogen	Parenteral	IV, SQ	Treatment of anemia due to kidney failure or cancer	Three times weekly	1000U, 2000U, 3000U, 4000U, 5000U, 6000U, 8000U, 10,000U, 20,000U, 30,000U, 40,000U
factor VIIa recombinant	NovoSeven	Parenteral	IV	Treatment of bleeding due to hemophilia	PRN	1mg, 2mg, 5mg
multivitamin	Centrum	Tablet	Oral	Vitamin supplement	q.d.	N/A
multivitamin, prenatal	Primacare One	Tablet	Oral	Vitamin supplement	q.d.	N/A
drotrecogin alfa	Xigris	Parenteral	IV	Prevent blood clots during sepsis	Infusion	5mg, 20mg
thrombin	Thrombin-JMI	Topical	Topical	Temporary bleeding control	PRN	5000U, 20,000U
folic acid	Folvite	Tablet, parenteral	PO, IV, IM, SQ	Treatment of anemia due to folic acid deficiency	q.d.	400mcg, 1mg

Table 14-2. Common Chemotherapy Agents Used to Treat Certain Types of Cancer

Generic Name	Brand Name	Dosage Form	Route
anastrozole	Arimidex	Tablet	PO
bevacizumab	Avastin	Parenteral	IV
busulfan	Myleran	Tablet, parenteral	PO, IV
bleomycin	Blenoxane	Parenteral	IV, IM
bortezomib	Velcade	Parenteral	IV
carboplatin	Carboplatin	Parenteral	IV
cetuximab	Erbitux	Parenteral	IV
chlorambucil	Leukeran	Tablet	PO
cisplatin	Platinol	Parenteral	IV
cyclophosphamide	Cytoxan	Tablet, parenteral	PO, IV

(Continued)

Table 14-2. Common Chemotherapy Agents Used to Treat Certain Types of Cancer *(Continued)*

Generic Name	Brand Name	Dosage Form	Route
docetaxel	Taxotere	Parenteral	IV
doxorubicin	Adriamycin, Doxil	Parenteral	IV
exemestane	Aromasin	Tablet	PO
fludarabine phosphate	Fludara	Tablet, parenteral	PO, IV
fluorouracil	Adrucil	Parenteral	IV
gemcitabine	Gemzar	Parenteral	IV
goserelin	Zoladex	Parenteral	SQ
hydroxyurea	Droxia, Hydrea	Capsule	PO
irinotecan	Camptosar	Parenteral	IV
lenalidomide	Revlimid	Capsule	PO
letrozole	Femara	Tablet	PO
leuprolide	Lupron	Parenteral	IM, SQ
mechlorethamine	Mustargen	Parenteral	IV
melphalan	Alkeran	Tablet, parenteral	PO, IV
mercaptopurine	Purinethol	Tablet	PO
methotrexate	Methotrexate, Rheumatrex, Trexall	Tablet, parenteral	PO, IV
mitotane	Lysodren	Tablet	PO
oxaliplatin	Eloxatin	Parenteral	IV
paclitaxel	Taxol	Parenteral	IV
pemetrexed	Alimta	Parenteral	IV
procarbazine	Matulane	Capsule	PO
rituximab	Rituxan	Parenteral	IV
tamoxifen	Nolvadex	Tablet	PO
trastuzumab	Herceptin	Parenteral	IV
vinblastine	Velban	Parenteral	IV
vincristine	Vincasar PFS	Parenteral	IV

Dosage Forms, Routes of Administration, and Usual Doses for Common Hematology and Oncology Medications

Many hematologic medications are available in oral form, allowing patients to take the medication on a continual basis at home. In some instances, such as with cyanocobalamin, a parenteral approach may be more convenient for the patient or may be the only method of administration possible while hospitalized. The nasal spray formulation of cyanocobalamin allows the patient to self-administer the medication and dose the medication only once weekly.

Medications used to treat cancer are often given parenterally. In some instances, the medications must infuse over a several hours, requiring that the patient either be hospitalized or go to an infusion center. In other instances, the patient may be able to take oral tablets or capsules from home. As noted earlier, it is also common to see combination therapy with medications used to treat cancer.

Common Side Effects of Hematology and Oncology Medications

Iron supplements, whether in the sulfate, gluconate, or fumarate form, may cause gastrointestinal side effects. Constipation is particularly common, as is nausea, stomach cramping, pain, and vomiting.

Medications used to treat cancer are known for strong and frequent side effects. Nausea, vomiting, and stomach upset are common with some agents, but less common with others. If nausea or vomiting is expected, a physician will likely prescribe an additional medication to combat these side effects. Other chemotherapy agents may cause a patient's hair to fall out. Injection site pain, fever, and blood disorders may develop as well. Patients taking medications to treat cancer will likely also be more susceptible to infections, so health care practitioners may pay special attention to signs and symptoms of infections during routine visits.

Terminology and Common Abbreviations Used with Hematology and Oncology Medications

See Table 2-1, page 13, for abbreviations.

What's in a Name?

Table 14-3.	Examples of USAN Stems for Hematology and Oncology Medications	
Stem	**Description**	**Example**
-mestane	Antineoplastics (aromatase inhibitors)	exemestane
-cogin	Blood coagulation cascade inhibitor	drotrecogin alfa
-poetin	Erythropoietins	epoetin alfa
-grastim	Granulocyte-colony stimulating factors (G-CSF)	filgrastim
-relin	Prehormones or hormone-release stimulating peptides	goserelin

Sample Prescription for Hematology and Oncology Medications

DEA # BD0000000

John Doe, M.D.
123 Any Street
Any Town, Any State 00000
Tel. (123) 456-7890   Fax. (123) 456-1234

NAME *Sherry Reynolds*

ADDRESS *1998 Fenwick Ct.*

Rx   *Feosol 200mg #30*

Sig: *T I T PO QD*

_____   M.D.
J. Doe,
(Signature)

REFILL *NR*

This prescription should be interpreted as: Feosol (ferrous sulfate) 200mg. Take one tablet by mouth every day. Dispense 30 tablets with no refills.

Alternative Therapies for Hematology and Oncology Conditions

Few, if any, alternative therapies exist for blood issues, particularly clotting issues. However, when it comes to cancer chemotherapy, many additional therapies exist that complement the treatment. For instance, a patient may take a portable music device with relaxing music to the infusion center, or a book to read as a distraction from the side effects of the medications. Other relaxation and stress-relief techniques may be helpful to avoid or minimize some side effects.

Chapter Summary !

Oncology treatments are used to treat cancer and are commonly delivered parenterally. However, some oral cancer treatments are also used. Hematologic conditions—that is, conditions affecting the blood such as anemia—may be treated with long-term oral medications. Sometimes parenteral medications in the hospital can be necessary or beneficial to the patient. Specific considerations include the following:

℞ Many oncology treatments are delivered in a regimen of two or more medications at once. Because treatments for cancer are constantly evolving and are patient-specific, treatment regimens may be quite different from one patient to the next

℞ Anemias may have a genetic component, be related to vitamin deficiencies, or be related to cancer chemotherapy. The treatment for each cause may be different

A physician or pharmacist should carefully monitor hematologic and oncologic treatments not only for how well the treatment is working but also to manage any side effects that may occur.

STUDENT NAME _____

DATE _____   INSTRUCTOR'S NAME _____

ANATOMY, PHYSIOLOGY, AND PHARMACOLOGY QUESTIONS

Identify whether the following questions are true or false (circle one).

1. Anemias can be caused by iron deficiency, vitamin B_{12} deficiency, or folic acid deficiency, among other causes.

   TRUE   FALSE

2. Red blood cell deficiency can be caused by some forms of cancer.

   TRUE   FALSE

3. Cancer chemotherapy can be used with radiation and/or surgery.

   TRUE   FALSE

4. Chemotherapy agents are usually stored and handled in the same way as other legend drugs.

   TRUE   FALSE

5. Multivitamins can have different formulations for different purposes, such as prenatal vitamins for pregnant women.

   TRUE   FALSE

MEDICATION QUESTIONS

Match the following brand-name products with their generic names

1. _____ Neupogen
2. _____ NovoSeven
3. _____ Slow Fe
4. _____ Cyklokapron
5. _____ Neulasta
6. _____ Ferretts
7. _____ Niferex
8. _____ Epogen

A. iron polysaccharide
B. epoetin alfa
C. filgrastim
D. ferrous sulfate
E. pegfilgrastim
F. tranexamic acid
G. ferrous fumarate
H. factor VIIa recombinant

9. _____ Amicar

10. _____ Aranesp

11. _____ Folvite

12. _____ Centrum

13. _____ Fergon

14. _____ Mephyton

15. _____ Feosol

16. _____ Primacare One

A. ferrous gluconate

B. ferrous sulfate

C. aminocaproic acid

D. phytonadione

E. darbepoetin Alfa

F. multivitamin

G. multivitamin, prenatal

H. folic acid

17. _____ Alkeran

18. _____ Vincasar PFS

19. _____ Taxol

20. _____ Doxil

21. _____ Hydrea

22. _____ Zoladex

23. _____ Lysodren

24. _____ Myleran

A. doxorubicin

B. busulfan

C. melphalan

D. mitotane

E. paclitaxel

F. hydroxyurea

G. goserelin

H. vincristine

25. _____ Rheumatrex

26. _____ Adrucil

27. _____ Camptosar

28. _____ Taxotere

29. _____ Eloxatin

30. _____ Leukeran

31. _____ Purinethol

32. _____ Matulane

A. chlorambucil

B. oxaliplatin

C. irinotecan

D. methotrexate

E. docetaxel

F. mercaptopurine

G. fluorouracil

H. procarbazine

Hematology and Oncology Medications ✚

STUDENT NAME _____

DATE _____   INSTRUCTOR'S NAME _____

33.	_____ Avastin	A.	letrozole
34.	_____ Gemzar	B.	lenalidomide
35.	_____ Revlimid	C.	bevacizumab
36.	_____ Rituxan	D.	methotrexate
37.	_____ Femara	E.	hydroxyurea
38.	_____ Trexall	F.	rituximab
39.	_____ Droxia	G.	gemcitabine
40.	_____ Velcade	H.	bortezomib

41.	_____ Nolvadex	A.	cisplatin
42.	_____ Alimta	B.	methotrexate
43.	_____ Velban	C.	pemetrexed
44.	_____ Platinol	D.	doxorubicin
45.	_____ Trexall	E.	mechlorethamine
46.	_____ Adriamycin	F.	vinblastine
47.	_____ Fludara	G.	tamoxifen
48.	_____ Mustargen	H.	fludarabine phosphate

49.	_____ Erbitux	A.	cyclophosphamide
50.	_____ Aromasin	B.	bleomycin
51.	_____ Cytoxan	C.	anastrozole
52.	_____ Arimidex	D.	cetuximab
53.	_____ Blenoxane	E.	leuprolide
54.	_____ Herceptin	F.	trastuzumab
55.	_____ Lupron	G.	iron sucrose
56.	_____ Venofer	H.	exemestane

Select a common and appropriate frequency of administration (circle one).

1. Femiron	q.d.	q.week	PRN
2. darbepoetin Alfa	q.d.	q.week	PRN
3. Neupogen	q.d.	q.week	PRN
4. NovoSeven	q.d.	q.week	PRN
5. Fergon	q.d.	q.week	PRN

Identify whether the following are available parenterally, orally, or both (circle one).

1. Cyklokapron	Parenteral	Oral	Both
2. Phytonadione	Parenteral	Oral	Both
3. Xigris	Parenteral	Oral	Both
4. Niferex	Parenteral	Oral	Both
5. filgrastim	Parenteral	Oral	Both
6. factor VIIa recombinant	Parenteral	Oral	Both
7. Venofer	Parenteral	Oral	Both
8. Amicar	Parenteral	Oral	Both
9. Fergon	Parenteral	Oral	Both
10. Aranesp	Parenteral	Oral	Both

Select the appropriate main use/drug class (circle one).

1. Adrucil	Anemia	Cancer
2. Arimidex	Anemia	Cancer
3. Femiron	Anemia	Cancer
4. bevacizumab	Anemia	Cancer
5. filgrastim	Anemia	Cancer
6. Epogen	Anemia	Cancer
7. oxaliplatin	Anemia	Cancer
8. gemcitabine	Anemia	Cancer
9. Aranesp	Anemia	Cancer
10. Niferex	Anemia	Cancer
11. mechlorethamine	Anemia	Cancer
12. Revlimid	Anemia	Cancer
13. Fergon	Anemia	Cancer
14. Slow Fe	Anemia	Cancer
15. Herceptin	Anemia	Cancer

STUDENT NAME _____

DATE _____   INSTRUCTOR'S NAME _____

Identify whether the following questions are true or false (circle one).

1. Carboplatin is used parenterally to treat certain types of cancers.
   TRUE   FALSE

2. Vincristine is given orally.
   TRUE   FALSE

3. Epogen is given once weekly.
   TRUE   FALSE

4. Neulasta is given to treat a low white blood cell count due to cancer.
   TRUE   FALSE

5. Arimidex is given orally for the treatment of cancer.
   TRUE   FALSE

6. Doxorubicin is given orally.
   TRUE   FALSE

7. Niferex is given parenterally.
   TRUE   FALSE

8. Rheumatrex and Trexall are brand names for methotrexate.
   TRUE   FALSE

9. Melphalan is given both orally and parenterally.
   TRUE   FALSE

10. Drotrecogin alfa is used to treat cancer.
    TRUE   FALSE

Select the best available answer for the following questions.

1. Goserelin is used to _____.

   a. treat a low white blood cell count
   b. treat anemia
   c. control bleeding
   d. treat cancer

2. Slow FE and Fer-In-Sol are both brand names for _____.

   a. ferrous sulfate
   b. ferrous gluconate
   c. ferrous fumarate
   d. phytonadione

3. Cyklokapron is used to _____.

   a. treat hemophilia
   b. treat iron deficiency anemia
   c. reduce blood loss in surgery
   d. treat low white blood cell count

4. The brand name for filgrastim is _____, and it is used to _____.

   a. Neupogen, treat a low white blood cell count
   b. Epogen, treat anemia
   c. Neupogen, treat anemia
   d. Epogen, treat a low white blood cell count

5. Which of the following are used to treat cancer? _____

   a. doxorubicin
   b. tranexamic acid
   c. phytonadione
   d. thrombin

6. Chlorambucil is used to _____.

   a. treat anemia
   b. treat hemophilia
   c. treat cancer
   d. treat a low white blood cell count

7. Thrombin is used topically for _____.

   a. temporary bleeding control
   b. anemia
   c. cancer
   d. low white blood cell count

8. Xigris is used to _____.

   a. prevent blood clots during sepsis
   b. treat low white blood cell counts
   c. treat cancer
   d. treat anemia

STUDENT NAME _____

DATE _____ INSTRUCTOR'S NAME _____

9. Femara is the brand name of _____.

    a. gemcitabine
    b. melphalan
    c. cisplatin
    d. letrozole

10. The proper route of administration of Taxol is _____, and its generic name is _____.

    a. PO, docetaxel
    b. PO, paclitaxel
    c. IV, docetaxel
    d. IV, paclitaxel

11. What do Aranesp and Velban have in common? _____

    a. Both treat cancer
    b. Both are given IV
    c. Both are given PO
    d. Both treat anemia

12. Phytonadione is given to _____.

    a. prevent bleeding
    b. treat cancer
    c. treat anemia
    d. treat hemophilia

14. EXERCISES

DISCUSSION AND CRITICAL THINKING QUESTIONS

1. How are chemotherapy medications handled and stored in most pharmacies?

_____

_____

_____

_____

2. Which side effects of cancer chemotherapy may require additional medications?

_____

_____

_____

_____

_____

3. Why do community pharmacies not have many chemotherapy medications?

_____

_____

_____

_____

_____

STUDENT NAME _____

DATE _____   INSTRUCTOR'S NAME _____

SAMPLE PRESCRIPTIONS:

DEA # BD0000000

John Doe, M.D.
123 Any Street
Any Town, Any State 00000
Tel. (123) 456-7890   Fax. (123) 456-1234

NAME   *Betty Straw*

ADDRESS   *824 Lima Ave.*

R_X   *Aromasin 25mg #30*

Sig: *T 1 T PO QD*

_____   *J. Doe,*   M.D.
(Signature)

REFILL   *NR* _____

NDC 0009-7663-04

30 Tablets   Rx only

Aromasin® ㉕
exemestane tablets

25 mg

Distributed by
Pfizer **Pharmacia & Upjohn Co**
Division of Pfizer Inc, NY, NY 10017

---

1. What is the generic name for Aromasin?

   _____

   _____

2. How would you translate the Sig code into plain English so that the patient could understand the directions for use?

   _____

   _____

   _____

3. How many refills are given on this prescription?

_____

_____

_____

_____

4. What common condition(s) does this medication treat?

_____

_____

_____

_____

STUDENT NAME _____

DATE _____ INSTRUCTOR'S NAME _____

DEA # BD0000000

John Doe, M.D.
123 Any Street
Any Town, Any State 00000
Tel. (123) 456-7890   Fax. (123) 456-1234

NAME _Kelly Barklington_____

ADDRESS _2650 Factory Ave._____

R*x*   Cyanocobalamin 250mcg #90

Sig: T I T PO QD

_____ J. Doe, _____ M.D.
              (Signature)

REFILL _NR_____

---

1. By what other name is cyanocobalamin known?

   _____

   _____

2. How would you translate the Sig code into plain English so that the patient could understand the directions for use?

   _____

   _____

   _____

   _____

3. How many refills are given on this prescription?

_____

_____

_____

_____

4. What is a common use for this medication?

_____

_____

_____

_____

Other Commonly Used Medications

15

KEY TERMS

Imaging agents

Immunizations

Inactivated vaccine

Live, attenuated vaccine

Transplant rejection

Vaccination

Vaccines

LEARNING OBJECTIVES

After completing this chapter, the student will be able to:

1. List two drugs used to promote hair growth

2. Describe when imaging agents are commonly used

3. Explain the terms *immunizations* and *vaccines*

4. Describe how vaccines work

5. Define the term *transplant rejection*

6. List three commonly used IV supplements

7. Identify available dosage forms for other commonly used medications encountered in this chapter

8. Identify routes of administration for other commonly used medications encountered in this chapter

9. Identify usual doses for other commonly used medications encountered in this chapter

10. List common side effects of other commonly used medications encountered in this chapter

11. List abbreviations for terms associated with use of medication therapy for other commonly used medications encountered in this chapter

Other Important Medications

When working as a pharmacy technician, you may encounter some medications that have not been included in the first 14 chapters of this book. This concluding chapter is intended to provide you with information about these other important drugs. Medications covered in this chapter include immunizations, drugs used to treat hair loss, imaging agents, and immunosuppressant drugs used for organ transplant patients.

Knowing the following terms will be helpful as you learn about these other commonly used medications.

Imaging agents: Medications that are administered to improve the visibility of body structures for imaging diagnostic tests, such as X-rays and CT scans

Immunization: The process of administering a vaccine to protect against a disease (This term is often used interchangeably with the term *vaccination*)

Inactivated vaccine: A killed vaccine that is given by injection into the muscle

Live, attenuated vaccine: A weakened influenza vaccine that is sprayed into the nostrils

Transplant rejection: The body's attack of a transplanted organ by the immune system of the person who receives the organ

Vaccination: The process of administering a vaccine to protect against a disease (This term is often used interchangeably with the term *immunization*)

Vaccines: Medications that work by helping the immune system to produce substances that naturally fight germs

Primer on Pharmacologic Actions of Other Commonly Used Medications

In the past 30 years, medications have been developed to promote hair growth. Finasteride (Propecia) is an example of a drug used to treat male pattern hair loss. Finasteride works by blocking the production of a male hormone in the scalp that stops hair growth. Minoxidil (Rogaine) is another drug used to stimulate hair growth.

Imaging agents known as radiocontrast agents are administered to improve the visibility of body structures for diagnostic tests such as X-ray imaging and CT scans. Iohexol (Omnipaque) is an example of an imaging agent.

Immunizations are given to adults and children to help prevent them from getting certain diseases that are caused by germs. They are commonly administered for diseases such as influenza, hepatitis A, hepatitis B, diphtheria, tetanus, and pertussis, among others. Immunizations are also known as vaccinations. Vaccines work by helping the immune system to produce substances that naturally fight germs, so when a vaccine is given to a healthy person, the immune system responds by building immunity to the germ. The most commonly administered vaccine in community pharmacies is the influenza vaccine, and there are two types:

℞ Inactivated (killed) vaccine is given by injection into the muscle

℞ Live, attenuated (weakened) influenza vaccine is sprayed into the nostrils

Influenza viruses constantly change, and the influenza vaccine is changed each year so that the viruses in the vaccine cover the types of flu that are most likely to cause sickness that year.

In recent years, organ transplantation has become more commonplace, especially for kidney, liver, and heart transplants. One complication of organ transplantation is transplant rejection. Transplant rejection is the body's attack of the transplanted organ by the immune system of the person who received the organ. Medications that decrease the activity of the immune system are used to prevent transplant rejection, and often numerous medications are needed in combination to prevent rejection. Cyclosporine (Sandimmune) is an example of a medication used with other medications to prevent transplant rejection. It works by suppressing the immune system.

Solutions of supplements are sometimes added to IVs to maintain proper electrolyte and mineral balance. Additionally, some supplements are administered for specific therapeutic indications. Examples of the supplements are calcium chloride, calcium gluconate, magnesium chloride, potassium phosphate, potassium acetate, sodium bicarbonate, and sodium chloride.

Some additional commonly used medications and their uses are listed in Table 15-1.

Table 15-1. Other Commonly Used Medications and Their Uses

Generic Name	Brand Name	Dosage Form	Route	Common Use	Common Frequency	Common Strengths
finasteride	Propecia	Tablet	PO	Hair growth	q.d.	1mg
minoxidil	Rogaine	Liquid	Topical	Hair growth	b.i.d.	2%, 5%
adenosine	Adenoscan	Parenteral	IV	Imaging agent	Infusion	3mg/ml
gadopentetate dimeglumine	Magnevist	Parenteral	IV	Imaging agent	Infusion	469.01mg/ml
iodixanol	Visipaque	Parenteral	IV	Imaging agent	Infusion	550mg/ml, 652mg/ml
iohexol	Omnipaque	Parenteral	IV	Imaging agent	Infusion	302mg/ml, 388mg/ml, 518mg/ml, 647mg/ml, 755mg/ml
ioversol	Optiray	Parenteral	IV	Imaging agent	Infusion	34%, 51%, 64%, 68%, 74%
iopamidol	Isovue	Parenteral	IV	Imaging agent	Infusion	51%, 61%, 76%
antithymocyte globulin	Thymoglobulin	Parenteral	IV	Immunosuppressant, organ rejection	Infusion for 1-2 weeks	25mg
cyclosporine	Neoral, Gengraf, Sandimmune	Capsule, liquid, parenteral	PO, IV	Immunosuppressant, organ rejection	b.i.d.	25mg, 50mg, 100mg, 50mg/ml, 100mg/ml
mycophenolate	CellCept, Myfortic	Tablet, capsule, liquid, parenteral	PO, IV	Immunosuppressant, organ rejection	b.i.d.	180mg, 250mg, 360mg, 500mg, 200mg/ml
sirolimus	Rapamune	Tablet, liquid	PO	Immunosuppressant, organ rejection	q.d.	1mg, 2mg
tacrolimus	Prograf	Capsule, parenteral	PO, IV	Immunosuppressant, organ rejection	b.i.d.	0.5mg, 1mg, 5mg
onabotulinum-toxin A	Botox	Parenteral	IM	Migraine headaches, spasticity, cosmetic	PRN	50 units, 100 units, 200 units

Table 15-2. Some Vaccines You Should Know

Vaccine	Common Abbreviation(s)	Common Use
Diphtheria, tetanus, pertussis	DTaP, DT, Tdap, Td	Preventing diphtheria, tetanus, and pertussis
Haemophilus influenzae type b	Hib	Preventing *Haemophilus influenzae* type b
Hepatitis A	HepA	Preventing hepatitis a
Hepatitis B	HepB	Preventing hepatitis b
Human papillomavirus	HPV	
Influenza, live attenuated	LAIV	Preventing selected strains of influenza
Influenza, trivalent inactivated	TIV	Preventing selected strains of influenza
Measles, mumps, rubella	MMR	Preventing measles, mumps and rubella
Meningococcal, conjugated	MCV4	Preventing four strains (or types) of bacterial meningitis caused by the bacteria *Neisseria meningitidis*
Pneumococcal conjugate	PCV	Preventing *Streptococcus pneumoniae* infection
Pneumococcal polysaccharide	PPV	Preventing *Streptococcus pneumoniae* infection
Varicella	Var	Preventing chicken pox

Table 15-3. Some Combination Vaccines You Should Know

Brand Name	Vaccines
Comvax	Hib+HepB
Pediarix	DTaP+HepB+IPV
ProQuad	MMR+Var
Trihibit	DTaP+Hib

Table 15-4. Some IV Supplements You Should Know

Common Name
Calcium chloride
Calcium gluconate
Magnesium chloride
Potassium phosphate
Potassium acetate
Sodium bicarbonate
Sodium chloride

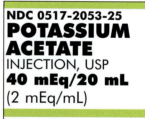

NDC 0517-2053-25
POTASSIUM ACETATE
INJECTION, USP
40 mEq/20 mL
(2 mEq/mL)

20 mL
SINGLE DOSE VIAL
FOR IV USE AFTER DILUTION
Rx Only
AMERICAN REGENT, INC.
SHIRLEY, NY 11967

Each mL contains: Potassium Acetate (Anhydrous) 196 mg (2 mEq), Water for Injection q.s. pH adjusted with Acetic Acid.
4 mOsmol/mL
Contains no more than 25,000 mcg/L of aluminum.
WARNING: DISCARD UNUSED PORTION. USE ONLY IF SOLUTION IS CLEAR.
Store at 20°-25°C (68°-77°F) (See USP Controlled Room Temperature). Directions for Use: See Package Insert.
Rev. 11/05

Dosage Forms, Routes of Administration, and Usual Doses for Other Commonly Used Medications

Vaccines are most often given as injections, because the natural defenses of the human gastrointestinal system will inactivate a vaccine. The influenza vaccine can be given as a nasal spray to some patients, particularly if they are healthy and at low risk for complications. Imaging agents are often given parenterally either before or during an imaging procedure.

Minoxidil, a medication developed to regrow hair, can be applied topically to the site where hair growth is desired. Alternatively, finasteride is a medication used for hair growth that is given orally.

Common Side Effects of Other Commonly Used Medications

Most immunizations, because they are given by injection, may cause some redness and irritation at the injection site. Some general discomfort may result for a day or two as the immunization works. In many cases, such as with the injected influenza virus, it is not possible to get the flu from the vaccine. Side effects with imaging agents are uncommon, although injection site reactions may occur. Minoxidil may cause nausea and vomiting, and finasteride can cause sexual side effects.

Terminology and Common Abbreviations Used with Other Commonly Used Medications

See Table 2-1, page 13, for abbreviations.

What's in a Name?

Table 15-5. Examples of USAN Stems for Other Commonly Used Medications		
Stem	**Description**	**Example**
-steride	Testosterone reductase inhibitors	finasteride
-imus	Immunosuppressives	tacrolimus

Sample Prescription for Other Commonly Used Medications

DEA # BD0000000

John Doe, M.D.
123 Any Street
Any Town, Any State 00000
Tel. (123) 456-7890   Fax. (123) 456-1234

NAME _Janet Smith_

ADDRESS _111 N. Main St._

℞   Propecia 1mg #30

Sig: T I T PO QD

_____J. Doe_____ M.D.
(Signature)

REFILL _Rfx2_

This prescription should be interpreted as: Propecia (finasteride) 1mg. Take one tablet by mouth every day. Dispense 30 tablets with two refills.

Technician Tip

Women of childbearing age should not touch or handle broken tablets of finasteride because the medication can be absorbed through the skin and may harm a developing fetus. If you are concerned about handling finasteride, talk with your pharmacist. ℞

Alternative Therapies for Other Commonly Used Medications

Few alternative therapies exist that are comparable to immunizations. Diseases targeted with immunizations are difficult to treat or can be problematic for the patient. If a patient chooses to forgo immunization, reducing or eliminating exposure to people with the diseases that were not immunized against could help reduce the risk of contracting that disease.

Chapter Summary !

Not all commonly used medications fit well into general classes. However, technicians should be familiar with a few other smaller categories of medications.

℞ Imaging agents are used with several types of scans in the hospital to help health care professionals better understand some conditions. Many imaging agents are given parenterally

℞ Following organ transplant, medications may be necessary to prevent the body from attacking the new organ. Oral and parenteral medications are available to prevent organ rejection

Pharmacists, particularly in the outpatient setting, are becoming more and more involved in the delivery of immunizations. Immunizations are often given parenterally and may be recommended based on a patient's age or other health conditions.

STUDENT NAME _____

DATE _____   INSTRUCTOR'S NAME _____

Match the following brand-name products with their generic names.

1. _____ Optiray	A. iopamidol
2. _____ Propecia	B. mycophenolate
3. _____ Rogaine	C. finasteride
4. _____ Visipaque	D. cyclosporine
5. _____ Neoral	E. Iohexol
6. _____ Omnipaque	F. Ioversol
7. _____ Myfortic	G. minoxidil
8. _____ Isovue	H. iodixanol

9. _____ Sandimmune	A. mycophenolate
10. _____ Rapamune	B. cyclosporine
11. _____ Adenoscan	C. adenosine
12. _____ CellCept	D. tacrolimus
13. _____ Thymoglobulin	E. gadopentetate dimeglumine
14. _____ Magnevist	F. antithymocyte globulin
15. _____ Prograf	G. sirolimus

Match the following vaccine to its abbreviation.

1. _____ Measles, mumps, rubella	A. LAIV
2. _____ Influenza, trivalent inactivated	B. Var
3. _____ Tetanus, diphtheria, and pertussis	C. MCV4
4. _____ Varicella	D. DTaP + Hib
5. _____ Comvax	E. MMR
6. _____ Influenza, live attenuated	F. Hib + HepB
7. _____ Meningococcal, conjugated	G. Tdap
8. _____ TriHIBit	H. TIV

9. _____ Hepatitis A

10. _____ Haemophilus influenzae type b

11. _____ Pediarix

12. _____ Pneumococcal conjugate

13. _____ Pneumococcal polysaccharide

14. _____ Hepatitis B

15. _____ Diphtheria, tetanus, and pertussis

16. _____ ProQuad

A. DTaP + HepB + IPV

B. PPV

C. MMR + Var

D. DTaP

E. HepA

F. Hib

G. HepB

H. PCV

Select a common and appropriate frequency of administration (circle one).

1. Prograf	q.d.	b.i.d.	Infusion
2. Magnevist	q.d.	b.i.d.	Infusion
3. Iohexol	q.d.	b.i.d.	Infusion
4. Rogaine	q.d.	b.i.d.	Infusion
5. Sirolimus	q.d.	b.i.d.	Infusion
6. Myfortic	q.d.	b.i.d.	Infusion
7. Optiray	q.d.	b.i.d.	Infusion
8. Finasteride	q.d.	b.i.d.	Infusion
9. Gengraf	q.d.	b.i.d.	Infusion
10. Adenosine	q.d.	b.i.d.	Infusion

Identify whether the following are available parenterally, orally, or both (circle one).

1. Cyclosporine	Parenteral	Oral	Both
2. Iopamidol	Parenteral	Oral	Both
3. Propecia	Parenteral	Oral	Both
4. Tacrolimus	Parenteral	Oral	Both
5. Sirolimus	Parenteral	Oral	Both
6. Iodixanol	Parenteral	Oral	Both
7. Adenosine	Parenteral	Oral	Both
8. Mycophenolate	Parenteral	Oral	Both
9. Magnevist	Parenteral	Oral	Both
10. Ioversol	Parenteral	Oral	Both

STUDENT NAME _____

DATE _____ INSTRUCTOR'S NAME _____

Select the appropriate main use/drug class (circle one).

1. Thymoglobulin   Imaging   Organ rejection

2. Isovue   Imaging   Organ rejection

3. Sandimmune   Imaging   Organ rejection

4. Prograf   Imaging   Organ rejection

5. Visipaque   Imaging   Organ rejection

6. Iohexol   Imaging   Organ rejection

7. Neoral   Imaging   Organ rejection

8. Sirolimus   Imaging   Organ rejection

9. Adenoscan   Imaging   Organ rejection

10. Ioversol   Imaging   Organ rejection

Identify if the following questions are true or false (circle one).

1. Minoxidil and finasteride are both applied topically.

   TRUE   FALSE

2. Isovue is a brand name of adenosine.

   TRUE   FALSE

3. Mycophenolate is used to prevent organ rejection.

   TRUE   FALSE

4. Prograf is dosed once daily, whereas Rapamune is dosed twice daily.

   TRUE   FALSE

5. Thymoglobulin is only available parenterally.

   TRUE   FALSE

6. Optiray and Omnipaque are both brand names for iopamidol.

   TRUE   FALSE

7. Cyclosporine is the generic of both Gengraf and Sandimmune.

   TRUE   FALSE

8. Magnevist is used for hair growth.

   TRUE   FALSE

9. Visipaque is used as an imaging agent.

   TRUE   FALSE

10. Botox can be used for migraine headaches.

   TRUE   FALSE

Select a common strength for the following medications.

1. Cyclosporine

   a. 1mg
   b. 5mg
   c. 10mg
   d. 50mg

2. Finasteride

   a. 1mg
   b. 5mg
   c. 10mg
   d. 50mg

3. Tacrolimus

   a. 1mg
   b. 5mg
   c. 10mg
   d. 50mg

4. Mycophenolate

   a. 20mg
   b. 200mg
   c. 500mg
   d. 1000mg

5. Rogaine

   a. 5%
   b. 10%
   c. 15%
   d. 20%

6. Rapamune

   a. 1mg
   b. 5mg
   c. 10mg
   d. 50mg

Select the best available answer for the following questions.

1. Adenosine is considered _____.

   a. an immunosuppressant
   b. a treatment for organ rejection
   c. imaging agent
   d. hair growth agent

2. Sandimmune and Neoral are both brand names for _____.

   a. cyclosporine
   b. tacrolimus
   c. mycophenolate
   d. adenosine

3. The generic name for Propecia is _____, and it is used to _____.

   a. finasteride, prevent organ rejection
   b. finasteride, grow hair
   c. sirolimus, prevent organ rejection
   d. sirolimus, grow hair

4. Tacrolimus is generic for _____.

   a. Prograf
   b. Rapamune
   c. CellCept
   d. Gengraf

5. Minoxidil is used as _____.

   a. an immunosuppressant
   b. a treatment for organ rejection
   c. an imaging agent
   d. a hair growth agent

6. The generic name for Magnevist is _____.

   a. iodixanol
   b. gadopentetate dimeglumine
   c. antithymocyte globulin
   d. ioversol

7. The proper route of administration of Propecia is _____, and its generic name is _____.

   a. PO, finasteride
   b. PO, mycophenolate
   c. IV, finasteride
   d. IV, mycophenolate

8. What do ioversol and iohexol have in common? _____

   a. Both are imaging agents
   b. Both are given PO
   c. Both are applied topically
   d. Both are used to prevent organ rejection

9. CellCept and Myfortic both contain _____.

   a. tacrolimus
   b. cyclosporine
   c. mycophenolate
   d. sirolimus

10. The generic name of Rapamune is _____.

   a. sirolimus
   b. tacrolimus
   c. mycophenolate
   d. cyclosporine

STUDENT NAME _____

DATE _____ INSTRUCTOR'S NAME _____

SAMPLE PRESCRIPTIONS:

DEA # BD0000000

John Doe, M.D.
123 Any Street
Any Town, Any State 00000
Tel. (123) 456-7890   Fax. (123) 456-1234

NAME _Deena Ulysses_____

ADDRESS _678 Barrington Ct._____

Rx   Prograf 1mg #120

Sig: 2 T PO Q 12H

_____ J. Doe, _____ M.D.
(Signature)

REFILL _RFx3_____

1. What is the generic name for Prograf?

   _____

   _____

2. How would you translate the Sig code into plain English so that the patient could understand the directions for use?

   _____

   _____

   _____

3. How many refills are given on this prescription?

4. What other common strengths are available for Prograf oral tablets?

5. What is a common use for this medication?

STUDENT NAME _____

DATE _____ INSTRUCTOR'S NAME _____

DEA # BD0000000

John Doe, M.D.
123 Any Street
Any Town, Any State 00000
Tel. (123) 456-7890   Fax. (123) 456-1234

NAME _Robert Davidson_____

ADDRESS _2992 W. Pony Dr._____

Rx   Rogaine 2% #60ml

Sig: A UTD b.i.d.

_____ J. Doe, _____ M.D.
                  (Signature)

REFILL __NR_____

1. What is the generic name for Rogaine?

   _____

   _____

2. How would you translate the Sig code into plain English so that the patient could understand the directions for use?

   _____

   _____

   _____

3. How many refills are given on this prescription?

4. What common condition(s) does this medication treat?

Top 200 Brand Medications by Total Prescriptions

Rank	Medication	Chapter	Rank	Medication	Chapter	Rank	Medication	Chapter
1	Lipitor	5	31	Loestrin 24 Fe	11	61	Trilipix	5
2	Nexium	10	32	Vyvanse	8	62	Boniva	7
3	Plavix	5	33	Cialis	11	63	Avodart	11
4	Singulair	9	34	Suboxone	8	64	Glipizide XL	6
5	Lexapro	8	35	Aricept	8	65	Pristiq	8
6	Crestor	5	36	Benicar	5	66	Lidoderm	7
7	Synthroid	6	37	Januvia	6	67	Humalog	6
8	ProAir HFA	9	38	Lunesta	8	68	Vigamox	12
9	Advair Diskus	9	39	Ambien CR	8	69	Evista	7
10	Cymbalta	8	40	Niaspan	5	70	Flomax	11
11	Diovan	5	41	Xalatan	12	71	Chantix	8
12	Ventolin HFA	9	42	Levoxyl	6	72	Avalide	5
13	Diovan HCT	5	43	Benicar HCT	5	73	Protonix	10
14	Actos	6	44	Flovent HFA	9	74	Cozaar	5
15	Seroquel	8	45	NuvaRing	11	75	Vivelle-DOT	11
16	Levaquin	4	46	Lovaza	5	76	Vesicare	11
17	Lantus	6	47	Yaz	11	77	Prempro	11
18	Nasonex	12	48	NovoLog	6	78	Avelox	4
19	Viagra	11	49	Combivent	9	79	Dexilant/Kapidex	10
20	Lyrica	8	50	Namenda	8	80	Focalin XR	8
21	Celebrex	7	51	Detrol LA	11	81	Strattera	8
22	Concerta	8	52	Ortho Tri-Cyclen Lo	11	82	Xopenex HFA	9
23	Spiriva	9	53	Lantus SoloSTAR	6	83	Actonel	7
24	Premarin	11	54	Proventil HFA	9	84	Travatan Z	12
25	Effexor XR	8	55	Aciphex	10	85	Levemir	6
26	Tricor	5	56	Avapro	5	86	Lumigan	12
27	Zetia	5	57	Bystolic	5	87	Apri	11
28	Vytorin	5	58	Adderall XR	8	88	Levitra	11
29	OxyContin	7	59	Symbicort	9	89	Geodon	8
30	Abilify	8	60	Zyprexa	8	90	Micardis	5

(Continued)

Rank	Medication	Chapter	Rank	Medication	Chapter	Rank	Medication	Chapter
91	Exforge	5	128	Enablex	11	165	Doryx	4
92	Coumadin	5	129	Alphagan P	12	166	Differin	13
93	Janumet	6	130	Premarin vaginal	11	167	Clarinex	9
94	Ciprodex otic	12	131	Xopenex	9	168	Lotemax	12
95	Valtrex	4	132	Uroxatral	11	169	Astelin	12
96	Restasis	12	133	Asmanex	9	170	Transderm-Scop	15
97	Seroquel XR	8	134	Prevacid SoluTab	10	171	Humulin R	6
98	Micardis HCT	5	135	Moviprep	10	172	Levothroid	6
99	Actonel 150	7	136	Avandia	6	173	Advair HFA	9
100	Lotrel	5	137	Tekturna	5	174	Truvada	4
101	Tussionex	9	138	Propecia	15	175	Nuvigil	8
102	Prometrium	11	139	Ortho Evra	11	176	SF 5000 Plus	12
103	AndroGel	11	140	Solodyn	4	177	Yasmin	11
104	Kariva	11	141	Humulin 70/30	6	178	Bactroban	4
105	Patanol	12	142	Lanoxin	5	179	Ranexa	5
106	Voltaren gel	7	143	Asacol	10	180	Metadate CD	8
107	Hyzaar	5	144	Prevacid	10	181	Lamictal	8
108	Armour Thyroid	6	145	Atacand	5	182	Atrovent HFA	9
109	Nasacort AQ	12	146	Nitrostat	5	183	Simcor	5
110	Coreg CR	5	147	Combigan	12	184	Opana ER	7
111	Qvar	9	148	Halflytely	10	185	Rhinocort Aqua	12
112	Pataday	12	149	Relpax	8	186	Humalog Mix 75/25 Pen	6
113	Xyzal	9	150	Novolin 70/30	6	187	Carafate	10
114	Humulin N	6	151	Femara	14	188	Norvir	4
115	Vagifem	11	152	Tamiflu	4	189	Aspir-Low	5
116	Toprol XL	5	153	Zovirax topical	13	190	BenzaClin	13
117	Byetta	6	154	Lovenox	5	191	Skelaxin	7
118	Novolog Mix 70/30	6	155	Zymar	12	192	Duac Care System	13
119	Veramyst	12	156	Maxalt	8	193	Wellbutrin XL	8
120	Azor	5	157	Estrace vaginal	11	194	Arthrotec	7
121	Caduet	5	158	Exelon patch	8	195	Epiduo	13
122	Welchol	5	159	Intuniv	8	196	Pulmicort Flexhaler	9
123	Actoplus Met	6	160	Allegra-D 24 Hour	9	197	Omnaris	12
124	Provigil	8	161	Astepro 0.15%	12	198	Ortho Tri-Cyclen	11
125	Epipen	9	162	Maxalt MLT	8	199	Prandin	6
126	Aggrenox	5	163	Arimidex	14	200	Nevanac	12
127	Dilantin	8	164	Amitiza	10			

Source   Drugs.com, 2010. Available at http://drugtopics.modernmedicine.com/drugtopics/Chains+%26+Business/2010-Top-200-branded-drugs-by-total-prescriptions/ArticleStandard/Article/detail/727256?contextCategoryId=7604

Top 200 Generic Medications by Total Prescriptions

Rank	Medication	Chapter	Rank	Medication	Chapter	Rank	Medication	Chapter
1	Hydrocodone/acetaminophen	7	31	Cephalexin	4	61	Temazepam	8
2	Lisinopril	5	32	Trimethoprim/Sulfamethoxazole	4	62	Promethazine Tabs	9
3	Simvastatin	5	33	Fexofenadine	9	63	Glimepiride	6
4	Levothyroxine	6	34	Amoxicillin/clavulanate	4	64	Albuterol nebulizer solution	9
5	Amoxicillin	4	35	Ciprofloxacin hydrochloride	4	65	Tamsulosin hydrochloride	5
6	Amlodipine besylate	5	36	Pravastatin	5	66	Folic Acid	15
7	Azithromycin	4	37	Trazodone hydrochloride	8	67	Spironolactone	5
8	Alprazolam	8	38	Lovastatin	5	68	Amlodipine besylate benz	5
9	Hydrochlorothiazide	5	39	Triamterene w/hydrochlorothiazide	5	69	Amphetamine salt combination	8
10	Omeprazole	10	40	Carvedilol	5	70	Metformin hydrochloride ER	6
11	Metformin	6	41	Alendronate	7	71	Triamcinolone acetonide topical	13
12	Furosemide Oral	5	42	Ranitidine hydrochloride	10	72	Digoxin	5
13	Metoprolol Tartrate	5	43	Meloxicam	7	73	Lamotrigine	4
14	Atenolol	5	44	Diazepam	8	74	Cefdinir	4
15	Sertraline	12	45	Naproxen	7	75	Diltiazem CD	5
16	Metoprolol succinate	5	46	Propoxyphene-N/acetaminophen	7	76	Benazepril	5
17	Zolpidem Tartrate	8	47	Fluconazole	4	77	Topiramate	8
18	Oxycodone w/ acetaminophen	7	48	Methylprednisolone Tabs	9	78	Isosorbide mononitrate	5
19	Citalopram hydrobromide	8	49	Doxycycline	4	79	Ramipril	5
20	Gabapentin	8	50	Paroxetine	8	80	Risperidone	8
21	Ibuprofen	7	51	Oxycodone	8	81	Glyburide	6
22	Prednisone Oral	7	52	Clonidine	5	82	Penicillin V potassium	4
23	Tramadol	7	53	Amitriptyline	8	83	Lansoprazole	10
24	Lisinopril/hydrochlorothiazide	5	54	Allopurinol	15	84	Clindamycin Systemic	4
25	Fluoxetine	8	55	Enalapril	5	85	Bupropion XL	8
26	Lorazepam	8	56	Carisoprodol	7	86	Metronidazole Tabs	4
27	Warfarin	5	57	Acetaminophen w/Codeine	8	87	Glipizide	6
28	Clonazepam	8	58	Klor-Con	5	88	Divalproex sodium	8
29	Fluticasone Nasal	12	59	Pantoprazole	10	89	Tri-Sprintec	11
30	Cyclobenzaprine	7	60	Potassium Chloride	5	90	Losartan potassium	5

(Continued)

Rank	Medication	Chapter	Rank	Medication	Chapter	Rank	Medication	Chapter
91	Potassium chloride ER	5	128	Doxazosin	5	164	Venlafaxine	8
92	Phentermine	8	129	Methocarbamol	7	165	Oxybutynin chloride	11
93	Mirtazapine	8	130	Budeprion XL	8	166	Atenolol and chlorthalidone	5
94	Hydroxyzine	9	131	Clobetasol	13	167	Labetalol	5
95	Estradiol Oral	11	132	Sprintec	11	168	Cefuroxime Axetil	4
96	Valacyclovir hydrochloride	4	133	Nifedipine ER	5	169	Hydrocortisone Topical	13
97	Diclofenac Sodium SR	7	134	Aspirin, Enteric-Coated	5	170	Morphine Sulfate ER	7
98	Nitrofurantoin monohydrate macrocrystal	4	135	Fenofibrate	5	171	Fluocinonide	13
			136	Levetiracetam	5	172	Clindamycin Topical	13
99	Verapamil SR	5	137	Nitroglycerin	5	173	Nystatin Systemic	4
100	Venlafaxine ER	8	138	Chlorhexidine Gluconate	12	174	Prenatal 1+1	15
101	Mupirocin	4	139	Baclofen	7	175	Tramadol hydrochloride and acetaminophen	7
102	Buspirone HCl	8	140	Glipizide ER	6			
103	Gemfibrozil	5	141	Losartan potassium/ hydrochlorothiazide	5	176	Etodolac	7
104	Amphetamine salt combination SR	8				177	Indomethacin	7
105	Ondansetron	10	142	Endocet	7	178	Diphenoxylate w/ atropine	10
106	Famotidine	10	143	Dicyclomine HCl	10	179	Phenobarbital	8
107	Sumatriptan oral	8	144	Clarithromycin	4	180	Oxcarbazepine	8
108	Promethazine/Codeine	9	145	Bisoprolol and hydrochlorothiazide	5	181	Diltiazem	5
109	Propranolol HCl	5				182	Carbidopa/Levodopa	8
110	Terazosin	5	146	Glyburide/Metformin hydrochloride	6	183	Gianvi	11
111	Polyethylene Glycol	10				184	Amiodarone	5
112	Meclizine hydrochloride	10	147	Nabumetone	7	185	Felodipine ER	5
113	Acyclovir	4	148	Hydroxychloroquine	15	186	Cyanocobalamin	15
114	Fentanyl transdermal	8	149	Benztropine	8	187	Oxybutynin chloride ER	11
115	Methotrexate	14	150	Ropinirole hydrochloride	8	188	Promethazine and dextromethorphan	9
116	Finasteride	11	151	Minocycline	4			
117	Ocella	11	152	TriNessa	11	189	Terbinafine HCl	4
118	Ferrous Sulfate	15	153	Phenazopyridine hydrochloride	11	190	Fexofenadine and pseudoephedrine	9
119	Benzonatate	9	154	Phenytoin Sodium extended release	8			
120	Bupropion SR	8				191	Ondansetron ODT	10
121	Methadone HCl	7	155	Ketoconazole Topical	4	192	Hydromorphone HCl	7
122	Cheratussin AC	9	156	Hydroxyzine Pamoate	13	193	Diltiazem SR	5
123	Tizanidine HCl	7	157	Prednisolone sodium phosphate	9	194	Ergocalciferol	15
124	Quinapril	5	158	Hydralazine	5	195	Pramipexole	8
125	Butalbital/acetaminophen/ caffeine	8	159	Avaine	11	196	Medroxyprogesterone Tab	11
			160	Colchicine	7	197	Carbamazepine	8
126	Metoclopramide	10	161	Nortriptyline	8	198	Benazepril/HCTZ	5
127	Clotrimazole/betamethasone	13	162	Nystatin topical	4	199	Prednisolone acetate ophthalmic	12
			163	Bupropion ER	8	200	Lithium Carbonate	8

Source Drugs.com, 2010. Available at http://drugtopics.modernmedicine.com/drugtopics/Chains+%26+Business/2010-Top-200-generic-medications-by-total-prescriptions/ArticleStandard/Article/detail/727256?contextCategoryId=7604

Top 100 Over-the-Counter and Health and Beauty Care Products

Rank	Product	Rank	Product	Rank	Product
1	Private Label Cold/Allergy/Sinus Tablets/Packets	24	Private Label 1 & 2 Letter Vitamins	45	Osteo Bi Flex Mineral Supplements
2	Private Label Internal Analgesic Tablets	25	Airborne Cold/Allergy/Sinus Tablets/Packets	46	Motrin IB Internal Analgesic Tablets
3	Prilosec OTC Antacid Tablets	26	Tylenol PM Internal Analgesic Tablets	47	Private Label Weight Control/Nutritionals Liquid/Powder
4	Private Label Mineral Supplements	27	Nature Made 1 & 2 Letter Vitamins	48	LifeScan One Touch Glucose
5	Advil Internal Analgesic Tablets	28	Alli Weight Control Candy/Tablets	49	Zantac 150 Antacid Tablets
6	Tylenol Internal Analgesic Tablets	29	Crest Whitening Plus Scope Toothpaste	50	Commit Antismoking Tablets
7	Listerine Mouthwash/Dental Rinse	30	Mucinex Dm Cold/Allergy/Sinus Tablets/Packets	51	Private Label Anti Itch Treatments (Inc Calamine)
8	Private Label First Aid Ointments/Antiseptics	31	Sudafed PE Cold/Allergy/Sinus Tablets/Packets	52	NicoDerm CQ Antismoking Patch
9	Aleve Internal Analgesic Tablets	32	Private Label Cold/Allergy/Sinus Liquid/Powder	53	Crest Pro Health Toothpaste
10	Ensure Weight Control/Nutritionals Liquid/Powder	33	Private Label Nasal Spray/Drops/Inhaler	54	Abreva Lip Balm/Cold Sore Medication
11	Private Label Multi-Vitamins	34	Bayer Internal Analgesic Tablets	55	Children's Motrin Internal Analgesic Liquids
12	Nicorette Antismoking Gum	35	Centrum Silver Multi-Vitamins	56	Neosporin First Aid Ointments/Antiseptics
13	Private Label First Aid—Tape/Bandage/Gauze/Cotton	36	Colgate Total Toothpaste	57	Breathe Right Nasal Strips
14	Private Label Laxative Tablets	37	Vicks NyQuil Cold/Allergy/Sinus Liquid/Powder	58	Centrum Multi-Vitamins
15	Claritin Cold/Allergy/Sinus Tablets/Packets	38	Private Label Mouthwash/Dental Rinse	59	Imodium Ad Diarrhea Tablets
16	Claritin D Cold/Allergy/Sinus Tablets/Packets	39	Colgate Toothpaste	60	Crest Pro Health Mouthwash/Dental Rinse
17	Private Label Antacid Tablets	40	Tylenol Cold Cold/Allergy/Sinus Tablets/Packets	61	Theraflu Cold/Allergy/Sinus Tablets/Packets
18	Benadryl Cold/Allergy/Sinus Tablets/Packets	41	Alcon Opti Free Replenish Eye/Lens Care Solutions	62	Boost Weight Control/Nutritionals Liquid/Powder
19	Private Label Antismoking Gum	42	Band Aid First Aid - Tape/Bandage/Gauze/Cotton	63	Sensodyne Toothpaste
20	Mucinex Cold/Allergy/Sinus Tablets/Packets	43	Slim Fast Optima Weight Control/Nutritionals Liquid/Powder	64	Crest Whitestrips Tooth Bleaching/Whitening/Pwdr/Pl
21	Natures Bounty Mineral Supplements	44	Alcon Opti Free Express Eye/Lens Care Solutions	65	Excedrin Internal Analgesic Tablets
22	Crest Toothpaste			66	Icy Hot External Analgesics Rubs
23	Nature Made Mineral Supplements			67	Pepcid Ac Antacid Tablets

(Continued)

Rank	Product	Rank	Product	Rank	Product
68	Pepto Bismol Stomach Remedy Liquid/Powder	80	Tylenol Arthritis Internal Analgesic Tablets	92	Gas X Antacid Tablets
69	Metamucil Laxative/Stimulant Liquid/Powder/Oil	81	Monistat 1 Vaginal Treatments	93	Colgate Max Fresh Toothpaste
70	Bausch & Lomb Renu MultiPlus Eye/Lens Care Solutions	82	Tylenol Internal Analgesic Liquids	94	Private Label Antismoking Patch
71	Private Label Vaginal Treatments	83	First Response Pregnancy Test Kits	95	Vicks DayQuil Cold/Allergy/Sinus Tablets/Packets
72	Ensure Plus Weight Control/Nutritionals Liquid/Powder	84	Children's Tylenol Cold/Allergy/Sinus Liquid/Powder	96	Preparation H Hemorrhoidal Cream/Ointment/Spray
73	Alka Seltzer Plus Cold/Allergy/Sinus Tablets/Packets	85	One A Day Multi-Vitamins	97	Tylenol Sinus Cold/Allergy/Sinus Tablets/Packets
74	Private Label Manual Toothbrushes	86	Private Label Laxative/Stimulant Liquid/Powder/Oil	98	Claritin RediTabs Cold/Allergy/Sinus Tablets/Packets
75	Private Label Internal Analgesic Liquids	87	Ace Muscle/Body Support Devices	99	Excedrin Migraine Internal Analgesic Tablets
76	Zicam Nasal Spray/Drops/Inhaler	88	Fixodent Denture Adhesives	100	Monistat 3 Vaginal Treatments
77	Dulcolax Laxative Tablets	89	Crest Whitening Expressions Toothpaste		
78	Pepcid Complete Antacid Tablets	90	Slim Fast Optima Meal On The Go Weight Control/Nutritionals Liquid/Powder		
79	Therma Care Heat/Ice Packs	91	Scope Mouthwash/Dental Rinse		

Modified from Drug Topics, 2007. Available at http://drugtopics.modernmedicine.com/drugtopics/data/articlestandard//drugtopics/082008/492702/article.pdf to highlight the top medications.

Top 100 Hospital Medications by Total Prescriptions

Rank	Medication	Chapter	Rank	Medication	Chapter
1	Lovenox	5	31	Erbitux	14
2	Aranesp	5	32	Visipaque	15
3	Procrit	14	33	Primaxin	4
4	Revlimid	14	34	Simvastatin	5
5	Neulasta	14	35	Gammagard S/D	15
6	Remicade	14	36	Morphine Sulfate	7
7	Rituxan	14	37	Vancomycin HCl	4
8	Levaquin	4	38	Nexium	10
9	Avastin	14	39	Plavix	5
10	Zosyn	4	40	Zometa	7
11	Neupogen	14	41	Gamunex	14
12	Eloxatin	14	42	Camptosar	14
13	Diprivan	8	43	Risperdal	8
14	Propofol	8	44	Zyprexa	8
15	Omnipaque	15	45	Lupron Depot	14
16	Integrilin	5	46	Prevacid	10
17	Advair Diskus	9	47	Azithromycin	4
18	Sodium Chloride	5	48	Lipitor	5
19	Zyvox	4	49	Cubicin	4
20	Herceptin	14	50	Suprane	8
21	Protonix	10	51	Normal Saline Flush	15
22	Taxotere	14	52	Cardene IV	5
23	Angiomax	5	53	Adenoscan	5
24	Thrombin-JMI	5	54	Synagis	4
25	Cancidas	4	55	Ondansetron HCl	10
26	Ultane	8	56	Omeprazole	10
27	Seroquel	8	57	Ceftriaxone	4
28	Carimune NF Nanofiltered	4	58	Zemuron	8
29	Protonix IV	10	59	Alimta	14
30	Gemzar	14	60	Maxipime	4

(Continued)

Rank	Medication	Chapter	Rank	Medication	Chapter
61	NovoSeven	14	81	Ambisome	4
62	Lantus	6	82	Cipro IV	4
63	Optiray 320	15	83	Sandostatin	10
64	Activase	5	84	Keppra	8
65	Merrem	4	85	Optiray 350	15
66	Epogen	14	86	Albuminar-25	14
67	ReoPro	5	87	Botox	15
68	Isovue-300	15	88	Venofer	15
69	AcipHex	10	89	Paclitaxel	14
70	Fentanyl	7	90	Effexor XR	8
71	Combivent	9	91	Gabapentin	8
72	Zoladex	14	92	Aloxi	10
73	Abilify	8	93	Gardasil	15
74	Singulair	9	94	Trasylol	5
75	Enbrel	7	95	Xigris	4
76	Magnevist	15	96	Metformin HCl	6
77	Argatroban	5	97	Risperdal Consta	8
78	Thymoglobulin	14	98	Xopenex	9
79	Nexium IV	10	99	Prograf	15
80	Novolog	6	100	Isovue-370	15

Source: Online Pharmacy News, 2007. Available at http://www.thepharmacyone.com/news/pharmacy-facts/top-100-drugs-used-in-hospitals-in-2007/

Common Medications Requiring Refrigeration

Generic Name	Brand Name	Generic Name	Brand Name
Adalimumab	Humira	Insulin Detemir	Levemir
Amoxicillin, clavulanate*	Augmentin	Insulin Glargine	Lantus
Anakinra	Kineret	Insulin Glulisine	Apidra
Calcitonin	Fortical, Miacalcin	Insulin Lispro	Novolog
Cefaclor*	Ceclor	Latanoprost	Xalatan
Cefadroxil*	Duricef	Liotrix	Thyrolar
Cefuroxime*	Ceftin	Liraglutide	Victoza
Cephalexin*	Keflex	NPH Insulin	Humulin N
Clindamycin and benzoyl peroxide	Duac	NPH Insulin	Novolin N
Erythromycin and benzoyl peroxide	Benzamycin gel	Oseltamivir*	Tamiflu
Estradiol, norethindrone	CombiPatch	Penicillin V potassium*	V-Cillin K, Veetids
Etanercept	Enbrel	Pramlintide	Symlin
Etonogestrel and ethinyl estradiol vaginal ring	NuvaRing	Promethazine	Phenergan, Promethegan (suppositories)
Exenatide	Byetta	Regular Insulin	Humulin R
Formoterol	Foradil	Regular Insulin	Novolin R
Insulin Aspart	Humalog	Teriparatide	Forteo

This list is not intended to be all-inclusive, but simply a list of some common medications requiring refrigeration.

* Anti-infective requiring refrigeration after reconstitution only.

APPENDIX F

Common Herbal Supplements

Name	Possible Use(s)	Name	Possible Use(s)
Aloe vera	Topically for skin damage	Ginkgo biloba	Memory
Black cohosh	Arthritis	Hoodia	Weight loss
Echinacea	Prevent or treat colds, flu	Saw palmetto	Benign prostatic hyperplasia
Garlic	Cholesterol	St. John's wort	Depression
Ginger	Stomachache, nausea	Valerian root	Insomnia

APPENDIX G

Institute for Safe Medication Practices

ISMP's List of *Error-Prone Abbreviations, Symbols,* and *Dose Designations*

The abbreviations, symbols, and dose designations found in this table have been reported to ISMP through the ISMP Medication Error Reporting Program (MERP) as being frequently misinterpreted and involved in harmful medication errors. They should NEVER be used when communicating medical information. This includes internal communications, telephone/verbal prescriptions, computer-generated labels, labels for drug storage bins, medication administration records, as well as pharmacy and prescriber computer order entry screens.

The Joint Commission has established a National Patient Safety Goal that specifies that certain abbreviations must appear on an accredited organization's "do-not-use" list; we have highlighted these items with a double asterisk (**). However, we hope that you will consider others beyond the minimum Joint Commission requirements. By using and promoting safe practices and by educating one another about hazards, we can better protect our patients.

Abbreviations	Intended Meaning	Misinterpretation	Correction
µg	Microgram	Mistaken as "mg"	Use "mcg"
AD, AS, AU	Right ear, left ear, each ear	Mistaken as OD, OS, OU (right eye, left eye, each eye)	Use "right ear," "left ear," or "each ear"
OD, OS, OU	Right eye, left eye, each eye	Mistaken as AD, AS, AU (right ear, left ear, each ear)	Use "right eye," "left eye," or "each eye"
BT	Bedtime	Mistaken as "BID" (twice daily)	Use "bedtime"
cc	Cubic centimeters	Mistaken as "u" (units)	Use "mL"
D/C	Discharge or discontinue	Premature discontinuation of medications if D/C (intended to mean "discharge") has been misinterpreted as "discontinued" when followed by a list of discharge medications	Use "discharge" and "discontinue"
IJ	Injection	Mistaken as "IV" or "intrajugular"	Use "injection"
IN	Intranasal	Mistaken as "IM" or "IV"	Use "intranasal" or "NAS"
HS	Half-strength	Mistaken as bedtime	Use "half-strength" or "bedtime"
hs	At bedtime, hours of sleep	Mistaken as half-strength	
IU**	International unit	Mistaken as IV (intravenous) or 10 (ten)	Use "units"
o.d. or OD	Once daily	Mistaken as "right eye" (OD-oculus dexter), leading to oral liquid medications administered in the eye	Use "daily"
OJ	Orange juice	Mistaken as OD or OS (right or left eye); drugs meant to be diluted in orange juice may be given in the eye	Use "orange juice"
Per os	By mouth, orally	The "os" can be mistaken as "left eye" (OS-oculus sinister)	Use "PO," "by mouth," or "orally"
q.d. or QD**	Every day	Mistaken as q.i.d., especially if the period after the "q" or the tail of the "q" is misunderstood as an "i"	Use "daily"
qhs	Nightly at bedtime	Mistaken as "qhr" or every hour	Use "nightly"
qn	Nightly or at bedtime	Mistaken as "qh" (every hour)	Use "nightly" or "at bedtime"
q.o.d. or QOD**	Every other day	Mistaken as "q.d." (daily) or "q.i.d. (four times daily) if the "o" is poorly written	Use "every other day"
q1d	Daily	Mistaken as q.i.d. (four times daily)	Use "daily"
q6PM, etc.	Every evening at 6 PM	Mistaken as every 6 hours	Use "daily at 6 PM" or "6 PM daily"
SC, SQ, sub q	Subcutaneous	SC mistaken as SL (sublingual); SQ mistaken as "5 every;" the "q" in "sub q" has been mistaken as "every" (e.g., a heparin dose ordered "sub q 2 hours before surgery" misunderstood as every 2 hours before surgery)	Use "subcut" or "subcutaneously"
ss	Sliding scale (insulin) or ½ (apothecary)	Mistaken as "55"	Spell out "sliding scale;" use "one-half" or "½"
SSRI	Sliding scale regular insulin	Mistaken as selective-serotonin reuptake inhibitor	Spell out "sliding scale (insulin)"
SSI	Sliding scale insulin	Mistaken as Strong Solution of Iodine (Lugol's)	
i/d	One daily	Mistaken as "tid"	Use "1 daily"
TIW or tiw (also BIW or biw)	TIW: 3 times a week BIW: 2 times a week	TIW mistaken as "3 times a day" or "twice in a week" BIW mistaken ad "2 times a day"	Use "3 times weekly" Use "2 times weekly"
U or u**	Unit	Mistaken as the number 0 or 4, causing a 10-fold overdose or greater (e.g., 4U seen as "40" or 4u seen as "44"); mistaken as "cc" so dose given in volume instead of units (e.g., 4u seen as 4cc)	Use "unit"
UD	As directed ("ut dictum")	Mistaken as unit dose (e.g., diltiazem 125 mg IV infusion "UD" misinterpreted as meaning to give the entire infusion as a unit [bolus] dose)	Use "as directed"
Dose Designations and Other Information	Intended Meaning	Misinterpretation	Correction
Trailing zero after decimal point (e.g., 1.0 mg)**	1 mg	Mistaken as 10 mg if the decimal point is not seen	Do not use trailing zeros for doses expressed in whole numbers
No leading zero before a decimal point (e.g., .5 mg)**	0.5 mg	Mistaken as 5 mg if the decimal point is not seen	Use zero before a decimal point when the dose is less than a whole unit

© ISMP 2010

335

Institute for Safe Medication Practices

ISMP's List of *Error-Prone Abbreviations, Symbols,* and *Dose Designations* (continued)

Dose Designations and Other Information	Intended Meaning	Misinterpretation	Correction
Drug name and dose run together (especially problematic for drug names that end in "l" such as Inderal40 mg; Tegretol300 mg)	Inderal 40 mg Tegretol 300 mg	Mistaken as Inderal 140 mg Mistaken as Tegretol 1300 mg	Place adequate space between the drug name, dose, and unit of measure
Numerical dose and unit of measure run together (e.g., 10mg, 100mL)	10 mg 100 mL	The "m" is sometimes mistaken as a zero or two zeros, risking a 10- to 100-fold overdose	Place adequate space between the dose and unit of measure
Abbreviations such as mg. or mL. with a period following the abbreviation	mg mL	The period is unnecessary and could be mistaken as the number 1 if written poorly	Use mg, mL, etc. without a terminal period
Large doses without properly placed commas (e.g., 100000 units; 1000000 units)	100,000 units 1,000,000 units	100000 has been mistaken as 10,000 or 1,000,000; 1000000 has been mistaken as 100,000	Use commas for dosing units at or above 1,000, or use words such as 100 "thousand" or 1 "million" to improve readability
Drug Name Abbreviations	**Intended Meaning**	**Misinterpretation**	**Correction**
ARA A	vidarabine	Mistaken as cytarabine (ARA C)	Use complete drug name
AZT	zidovudine (Retrovir)	Mistaken as azathioprine or aztreonam	Use complete drug name
CPZ	Compazine (prochlorperazine)	Mistaken as chlorpromazine	Use complete drug name
DPT	Demerol-Phenergan-Thorazine	Mistaken as diphtheria-pertussis-tetanus (vaccine)	Use complete drug name
DTO	Diluted tincture of opium, or deodorized tincture of opium (Paregoric)	Mistaken as tincture of opium	Use complete drug name
HCl	hydrochloric acid or hydrochloride	Mistaken as potassium chloride (The "H" is misinterpreted as "K")	Use complete drug name unless expressed as a salt of a drug
HCT	hydrocortisone	Mistaken as hydrochlorothiazide	Use complete drug name
HCTZ	hydrochlorothiazide	Mistaken as hydrocortisone (seen as HCT250 mg)	Use complete drug name
MgSO4**	magnesium sulfate	Mistaken as morphine sulfate	Use complete drug name
MS, MSO4**	morphine sulfate	Mistaken as magnesium sulfate	Use complete drug name
MTX	methotrexate	Mistaken as mitoxantrone	Use complete drug name
PCA	procainamide	Mistaken as patient controlled analgesia	Use complete drug name
PTU	propylthiouracil	Mistaken as mercaptopurine	Use complete drug name
T3	Tylenol with codeine No. 3	Mistaken as liothyronine	Use complete drug name
TAC	triamcinolone	Mistaken as tetracaine, Adrenalin, cocaine	Use complete drug name
TNK	TNKase	Mistaken as "TPA"	Use complete drug name
ZnSO4	zinc sulfate	Mistaken as morphine sulfate	Use complete drug name
Stemmed Drug Names	**Intended Meaning**	**Misinterpretation**	**Correction**
"Nitro" drip	nitroglycerin infusion	Mistaken as sodium nitroprusside infusion	Use complete drug name
"Norflox"	norfloxacin	Mistaken as Norflex	Use complete drug name
"IV Vanc"	intravenous vancomycin	Mistaken as Invanz	Use complete drug name
Symbols	**Intended Meaning**	**Misinterpretation**	**Correction**
℥	Dram	Symbol for dram mistaken as "3"	Use the metric system
♏	Minim	Symbol for minim mistaken as "mL"	
x3d	For three days	Mistaken as "3 doses"	Use "for three days"
> and <	Greater than and less than	Mistaken as opposite of intended; mistakenly use incorrect symbol; "< 10" mistaken as "40"	Use "greater than" or "less than"
/ (slash mark)	Separates two doses or indicates "per"	Mistaken as the number 1 (e.g., "25 units/10 units" misread as "25 units and 110" units)	Use "per" rather than a slash mark to separate doses
@	At	Mistaken as "2"	Use "at"
&	And	Mistaken as "2"	Use "and"
+	Plus or and	Mistaken as "4"	Use "and"
°	Hour	Mistaken as a zero (e.g., q2° seen as q 20)	Use "hr," "h," or "hour"
Ø	zero, null sign	Mistaken as the numerals 4, 6, or 9	Use the number "0" or the word "zero"

© ISMP 2010

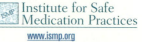

Institute for Safe Medication Practices

www.ismp.org

Answers to Practice Problems

CHAPTER 1

Matching
1. D
2. C
3. A
4. B
5. E
6. G
7. F
8. A
9. G
10. B
11. F
12. C
13. E
14. D
15. B
16. C
17. F
18. D
19. E
20. A

True/False
1. F
2. F
3. F
4. T
5. F
6. T
7. T
8. T
9. T
10. F

Multiple Choice
1. D
2. B
3. B
4. D
5. C
6. C
7. A
8. A
9. B
10. C

CHAPTER 2

Matching
1. E
2. G
3. H
4. B
5. A
6. C
7. F
8. D
9. B
10. G
11. E
12. D
13. H
14. C
15. F
16. A
17. E
18. D
19. C
20. B
21. F
22. G
23. H
24. A
25. G
26. F
27. H
28. D
29. E
30. A
31. C
32. B
33. C
34. B
35. G
36. F
37. H
38. E
39. D
40. A
41. E
42. A
43. D
44. B
45. H
46. G
47. C
48. F
49. B
50. H
51. C
52. A
53. D
54. G
55. F
56. E
57. D
58. G
59. A
60. B
61. C
62. H
63. E
64. F

True/False
1. F
2. T
3. F
4. T
5. F
6. T
7. F
8. F
9. T
10. F

Multiple Choice
1. B
2. C
3. B
4. A
5. B
6. D
7. A
8. C
9. A
10. B

CHAPTER 3

Matching
1. D
2. A
3. H
4. B
5. C
6. G
7. E
8. F
9. C
10. E
11. H
12. G
13. B
14. F
15. A
16. D
17. C
18. D
19. B
20. A

True/False
1. F
2. T
3. F
4. F
5. T

Multiple Choice
1. C
2. B
3. C
4. B
5. B
6. D
7. C
8. C
9. A
10. A

CHAPTER 4

Virus/Fungus
1. Virus
2. Fungus
3. Virus
4. Virus
5. Fungus

True/False
1. T
2. T
3. F
4. F
5. T

Matching
1. G
2. A
3. H
4. C
5. E
6. D
7. F
8. B
9. G
10. A
11. E
12. D
13. B
14. F
15. H
16. C
17. E
18. C
19. H
20. A
21. D
22. B
23. G
24. F
25. D
26. E
27. F
28. G
29. B
30. H
31. A
32. C
33. C
34. F
35. G
36. A

37. B
38. H
39. E
40. D
41. C
42. F
43. A
44. G
45. H
46. E
47. B
48. D

Parenteral/Oral/Both
1. Parenteral
2. Both
3. Both
4. Oral
5. Oral
6. Oral
7. Both
8. Both
9. Parenteral
10. Oral
11. Oral
12. Both
13. Both
14. Oral
15. Both
16. Parenteral
17. Oral
18. Parenteral
19. Oral
20. Oral

Antibiotic/Antiviral/ Antifungal/Anti-HIV
1. Antiviral
2. Antibiotic
3. Antibiotic
4. Anti-HIV
5. Antifungal
6. Anti-HIV
7. Antibiotic
8. Antibiotic
9. Antifungal
10. Antibiotic

True/False
1. F
2. T
3. T
4. T
5. F

Common Strength
1. C
2. D
3. D
4. C
5. C

6. A
7. A
8. A
9. D
10. C
11. C
12. B
13. A
14. D
15. C

Multiple Choice
1. B
2. A
3. C
4. C
5. D
6. C
7. D
8. B
9. A
10. C

Sample Prescription Cipro
1. Ciprofloxacin
2. Take one tablet by mouth twice daily for a sinus infection
3. One refill
4. 200mg, 250mg, 400mg, 750mg
5. Antibiotic
6. 5 days

Sample Prescription Diflucan
1. Fluconazole
2. Take one tablet by mouth now
3. No refills
4. 50mg, 100mg, 200mg
5. Antibiotic

CHAPTER 5

High blood pressure/High cholesterol
1. High blood pressure
2. High cholesterol
3. High blood pressure
4. High blood pressure
5. High cholesterol

True/False
1. T
2. T
3. F
4. F
5. T

Matching
1. F
2. G
3. A
4. G
5. E
6. C
7. B
8. D
9. D
10. A
11. F
12. H
13. C
14. G
15. B
16. E
17. B
18. A
19. E
20. F
21. C
22. H
23. D
24. G
25. H
26. D
27. A
28. E
29. C
30. B
31. H
32. G
33. B
34. E
35. C
36. H
37. A
38. G
39. F
40. D
41. B
42. D
43. G
44. A
45. H
46. C
47. E
48. F

Topical/Sublingual/ Oral/Parenteral
1. Sublingual
2. Parenteral
3. Oral
4. Parenteral
5. Oral
6. Oral
7. Topical
8. Oral

9. Parenteral
10. Oral

Parenteral/Oral/Both
1. Both
2. Oral
3. Parenteral
4. Parenteral
5. Oral
6. Both
7. Parenteral
8. Parenteral
9. Parenteral
10. Parenteral
11. Both
12. Oral
13. Both
14. Oral
15. Oral

Beta blocker/ ACE-inhibitor/ARB/ Diuretic/Calcium channel blocker
1. Beta blocker
2. ACE-Inhibitor
3. ARB
4. ACE-Inhibitor
5. ARB
6. Calcium channel blocker
7. Diuretic
8. Calcium channel blocker
9. Calcium channel blocker
10. Diuretic

True/False
1. T
2. F
3. T
4. T
5. F
6. T
7. F
8. T
9. F
10. F

Common Strength
1. C
2. A
3. D
4. B
5. C
6. C
7. B
8. A
9. D
10. A

11. C
12. C
13. A
14. B
15. B

Multiple Choice
1. B
2. B
3. D
4. A
5. A
6. A
7. D
8. A
9. A
10. A
11. C
12. B
13. B
14. A
15. C
16. D
17. D
18. C
19. C
20. B
21. C
22. A

Matching
1. D
2. C
3. J
4. F
5. G
6. H
7. A
8. B
9. E
10. I
11. K
12. L

Sample Prescription Caduet
1. Amlodipine and atorvastatin
2. Take one tablet by mouth daily
3. Eight refills
4. Hypertension and hyperlipidemia

Sample Prescription Coumadin
1. Warfarin
2. Take three tablets by mouth daily on Monday, Wednesday, and Friday, and take

four tablets by mouth daily on Tuesday, Thursday, Saturday, and Sunday.
3. One refill
4. 1mg, 2mg, 2.5mg, 3mg, 4mg, 5mg, 6mg, 7.5mg, 10mg
5. Prevent blood clot formation
6. 4 weeks or 28 days

CHAPTER 6

Matching
1. B
2. C
3. A
4. D

True/False
1. T
2. F
3. F
4. F
5. T

Matching
1. H
2. C
3. D
4. G
5. E
6. B
7. A
8. F
9. G
10. D
11. E
12. A
13. B
14. F
15. H
16. C
17. E
18. A
19. B
20. G
21. C
22. F
23. H
24. D

Parenteral/Oral/Both
1. Both
2. Parenteral
3. Parenteral
4. Oral
5. Oral
6. Parenteral
7. Parenteral

8. Oral
9. Both
10. Oral

Duration of Action
1. Long
2. Short
3. Rapid
4. Intermediate
5. Long
6. Intermediate
7. Rapid
8. Short
9. Rapid
10. Long
11. Intermediate
12. Rapid

True/False
1. T
2. T
3. F
4. F
5. F

Common Strength
1. D
2. A
3. C
4. B
5. C
6. B
7. C
8. C
9. D
10. B

Multiple Choice
1. A
2. C
3. C
4. A
5. A
6. A
7. A
8. D
9. B
10. B

Sample Prescription Lantus
1. Glargine
2. Parenteral – SQ
3. Inject 40 units every night at bedtime
4. Five refills
5. Long-acting insulin
6. 25 days

Sample Prescription Glyset
1. Miglitol

2. Take one tablet by mouth three times daily before meals
3. No refills
4. 25mg, 100mg
5. Diabetes
6. 30 days

Sample Prescription Humulin
1. Regular insulin
2. Inject 5 units three times daily before meals and using the sliding scale
3. Two refills
4. Diabetes
5. Short-acting insulin
6. 2 units
7. 5 units

CHAPTER 7

Osteoporosis/Pain
1. Pain
2. Osteoporosis
3. Pain
4. Osteoporosis
5. Osteoporosis

True/False
1. T
2. F
3. T
4. T
5. T

Matching
1. D
2. H
3. E
4. A
5. C
6. F
7. B
8. G
9. B
10. G
11. A
12. C
13. F
14. H
15. D
16. E
17. E
18. A
19. H
20. G
21. C
22. D
23. F

24. B
25. A
26. H
27. F
28. E
29. C
30. D
31. G
32. B
33. D
34. E
35. F
36. G
37. H
38. B
39. A
40. C
41. B
42. G
43. E
44. C
45. A
46. H
47. F
48. D
49. C
50. G
51. B
52. A
53. H
54. D
55. F
56. E

Frequency of Administration
1. q.d.
2. q.4-6h
3. b.i.d.
4. t.i.d.
5. t.i.d.
6. q.d.
7. q.d.
8. b.i.d.
9. q.4-6h
10. q.d.

DEA Control Schedule
1. C-II
2. C-III
3. C-II
4. C-II
5. C-II
6. C-III
7. C-IV
8. C-II
9. C-IV
10. C-III

Route of Administration
1. PO
2. SQ
3. PO
4. IN
5. PO
6. IV
7. SQ
8. PO
9. PO
10. SQ

Parenteral/Oral/Both
1. Both
2. Oral
3. Both
4. Both
5. Oral
6. Oral
7. Both
8. Oral
9. Both
10. Parenteral

Main Use/Drug Class
1. Pain
2. Osteoporosis
3. Relax muscles
4. Pain
5. Pain
6. Osteoporosis
7. Relax muscles
8. Osteoporosis
9. Pain
10. Pain

True/False
1. T
2. T
3. F
4. F
5. T
6. F
7. F
8. T
9. F
10. T

Common Strength
1. B
2. B
3. D
4. C
5. C
6. A
7. B
8. B
9. B
10. B
11. A

12. D
13. C
14. B
15. C

Multiple Choice
1. D
2. B
3. A
4. B
5. C
6. A
7. B
8. A
9. B
10. D
11. C
12. A
13. C
14. A
15. A

Sample Prescription Evista
1. Raloxifine
2. Take one tablet by mouth daily
3. Five refills
4. Osteoporosis in post-menopausal women

Sample Prescription Celebrex
1. Celecoxib
2. Take one tablet by mouth daily
3. One refill
4. 100mg
5. Treating pain and inflammation

Sample Prescription Toradol
1. Ketorolac
2. Take one tablet every six hours
3. No refills
4. Treating pain and inflammation

Sample Prescription Colcrys
1. Colchicine
2. Take two tablets by mouth as needed for gout pain. May take one tablet one hour after the first dose. Maximum 1.8mg per day
3. No refills
4. Treating gout

CHAPTER 8
PNS/CNS
1. PNS
2. CNS
3. CNS
4. PNS
5. PNS

True/False
1. F
2. T
3. F
4. T
5. F

Matching
1. A
2. C
3. G
4. H
5. B
6. F
7. E
8. D
9. G
10. F
11. H
12. D
13. B
14. A
15. E
16. C
17. B
18. E
19. G
20. A
21. F
22. C
23. D
24. H
25. C
26. D
27. F
28. G
29. H
30. A
31. E
32. B
33. D
34. C
35. F
36. E
37. G
38. A
39. H
40. B
41. D
42. B
43. G
44. F

45. A
46. C
47. H
48. E
49. B
50. H
51. E
52. D
53. G
54. A
55. C
56. F
57. H
58. F
59. A
60. E
61. D
62. C
63. G
64. B

Frequency of Administration
1. q.d.
2. b.i.d.
3. b.i.d.
4. q.d.
5. q.d.
6. q.d.
7. t.i.d.
8. b.i.d.
9. t.i.d.
10. q.d.

Route of Administration
1. PO
2. IV
3. PO
4. Transdermally
5. PO
6. IV
7. PO
8. Transdermally
9. IV
10. PO

Parenteral/Oral/Both
1. Both
2. Oral
3. Oral
4. Both
5. Oral
6. Both
7. Oral
8. Both
9. Oral
10. Both

Main Use/Drug Class
1. ADHD
2. Seizure Disorders

3. Seizure Disorders
4. Insomnia
5. ADHD
6. Insomnia
7. Seizure Disorders
8. ADHD
9. Seizure Disorders
10. Insomnia

Main Use/Drug Class
1. Parkinson's
2. Alzheimer's
3. Alzheimer's
4. Anxiety Disorders
5. Parkinson's
6. Anxiety Disorders
7. Parkinson's
8. Anxiety Disorders
9. Anxiety Disorders
10. Alzheimer's

True/False
1. T
2. F
3. T
4. F
5. T
6. T
7. F
8. T
9. F
10. T

Common Strength
1. C
2. D
3. D
4. A
5. A
6. A
7. B
8. A
9. A
10. D
11. D
12. B
13. C
14. B
15. A

Multiple Choice
1. B
2. C
3. D
4. A
5. D
6. B
7. B
8. A
9. C
10. C

11. A
12. B
13. B
14. D
15. A

Sample Prescription Focalin XR
1. Dexmethylphenidate
2. Take one tablet by mouth every morning
3. No refills
4. Yes, C-II
5. ADHD

Sample Prescription Suboxone
1. Buprenorphine and naloxone
2. Take one tablet by mouth daily
3. No refills
4. 2mg/0.5mg
5. To help treat addictions

Sample Prescription Zyprexa
1. Olanzapine
2. Take one tablet by mouth daily
3. Three refills
4. 2.5mg, 5mg, 7.5mg, 10mg, 15mg, 20mg
5. To treat schizophrenia

CHAPTER 9
Upper/Lower Respiratory Tract
1. Lower respiratory tract
2. Upper respiratory tract
3. Upper respiratory tract
4. Lower respiratory tract
5. Lower respiratory tract

True/False
1. T
2. F
3. T
4. F
5. F

Matching
1. G
2. C
3. A
4. D
5. F
6. H
7. E
8. B
9. A
10. C

11. F
12. B
13. D
14. G
15. H
16. E
17. E
18. D
19. A
20. H
21. B
22. F
23. C
24. G
25. C
26. F
27. D
28. A
29. B
30. H
31. G
32. E
33. F
34. B
35. C
36. E
37. A
38. H
39. D
40. G
41. A
42. E
43. B
44. G
45. C
46. F
47. D
48. H
49. C
50. E
51. D
52. A
53. F
54. H
55. G
56. B

Frequency of Administration
1. b.i.d.
2. q.d.
3. p.r.n.
4. q.4-6h
5. b.i.d.
6. q.d.
7. q.d.
8. b.i.d.
9. b.i.d.
10. q.4-6h

11. p.r.n.
12. q.4-6h
13. b.i.d.
14. b.i.d.
15. q.4-6h

Dosage Form
1. Inhaler
2. Nasal spray
3. Tablet
4. Inhaler
5. Liquid
6. Inhaler
7. Inhaler
8. Liquid
9. Nasal spray
10. Liquid

Parenteral/Oral/Both
1. Both
2. Oral
3. Parenteral
4. Both
5. Oral

Level of Control
1. OTC
2. C-V
3. Rx
4. Rx
5. OTC
6. OTC
7. C-V
8. Rx
9. OTC
10. Rx

Main Use/Drug Class
1. Decongestant
2. Asthma
3. Allergies
4. Asthma
5. Asthma
6. Decongestant
7. Allergies
8. Asthma
9. Allergies
10. Asthma
11. Multi-symptom cold relief
12. COPD
13. Cough
14. Multi-symptom cold relief
15. COPD
16. Cough
17. COPD
18. Cough
19. Multi-symptom cold relief
20. Cough

True/False
1. T
2. F
3. T
4. F
5. T
6. T
7. F
8. T
9. T
10. F

Common Strength
1. B
2. A
3. D
4. B
5. C
6. D
7. C
8. C
9. B
10. A
11. A
12. C
13. C
14. A
15. D

Multiple Choice
1. A
2. D
3. B
4. C
5. B
6. A
7. C
8. A
9. D
10. B
11. A
12. B
13. B
14. A
15. B

Sample Prescription Spiriva
1. Tiotropium
2. COPD
3. Inhale one puff daily
4. 30

Sample Prescription Robitussin AC
1. Guaifenesin and codeine
2. Cough suppression
3. Take one teaspoonful (5ml) by mouth every four to six hours as needed
4. 4 days
5. 4 ounces

Sample Prescription Zyrtec-D
1. Cetirizine 5mg and pseudoephedrine 120mg
2. Allergies
3. Take one tablet by mouth twice a day
4. 30 days

CHAPTER 10
True/False
1. F
2. F
3. T
4. T
5. T

Matching
1. H
2. F
3. G
4. B
5. C
6. A
7. E
8. D
9. B
10. D
11. G
12. H
13. A
14. F
15. C
16. E
17. C
18. A
19. G
20. F
21. D
22. G
23. E
24. B
25. F
26. B
27. A
28. G
29. C
30. H
31. E
32. D
33. E
34. D
35. B
36. C
37. F
38. H
39. A
40. G
41. C
42. A
43. H
44. G
45. B
46. F
47. D
48. E

Frequency of Administration
1. t.i.d.
2. q.i.d.
3. q.d.
4. q.i.d.
5. q.d.
6. b.i.d.
7. q.d.
8. q.i.d.
9. q.i.d.
10. q.d.

Dosage Form
1. Liquid
2. Tablet
3. Tablet
4. Liquid
5. Parenteral
6. Tablet
7. Liquid
8. Liquid
9. Tablet
10. Tablet

Parenteral/Oral/Both
1. Both
2. Oral
3. Oral
4. Both
5. Oral
6. Parenteral
7. Both
8. Oral
9. Both
10. Oral

OTC/Rx
1. OTC
2. OTC
3. Rx
4. OTC
5. Rx
6. OTC
7. RX
8. RX
9. OTC
10. OTC

Main Use/Drug Class
1. Nausea
2. Nausea
3. Heartburn
4. Diarrhea
5. Nausea
6. Heartburn
7. Nausea
8. Diarrhea
9. Heartburn
10. Diarrhea

True/False
1. T
2. F
3. T
4. F
5. F
6. T
7. T
8. T
9. F
10. F

Common Strength
1. D
2. A
3. D
4. D
5. B
6. A
7. C
8. A
9. C
10. B
11. A
12. B
13. B
14. A
15. C

Multiple Choice
1. B
2. B
3. C
4. A
5. C
6. C
7. C
8. D
9. A
10. B
11. C
12. C
13. A
14. B
15. D

Sample Prescription Lomotil
1. Diphenoxylate and atropine
2. Take one tablet by mouth four times daily as needed
3. No refills
4. Diarrhea
5. Liquid
6. 4 days
7. C-V
8. 5, because it is a controlled substance

Sample Prescription Xenical
1. Orlistat
2. Take one tablet by mouth three times daily before meals
3. One refill
4. Management of obesity
5. 30
6. Alli

Sample Prescription GoLytely
1. Polyethylene glycol electrolyte solution
2. Take 8 ounces by mouth every 10 minutes until gone
3. No refills
4. Cleansing the bowels before a gastrointestinal examination or surgery
5. 17

CHAPTER 11

Estrogen/ Progesterone/ Testosterone
1. Estrogen
2. Progesterone
3. Estrogen
4. Testosterone
5. Progesterone

True/False
1. F
2. T
3. F
4. F
5. T

Matching
1. B
2. F
3. H
4. A
5. E
6. D
7. C
8. G
9. C
10. B
11. E
12. A
13. H
14. G
15. D
16. F
17. D
18. C
19. F
20. H
21. B
22. E
23. G
24. A
25. H
26. G
27. F
28. B
29. D
30. C
31. A
32. E
33. F
34. C
35. G
36. E
37. D
38. B
39. A
40. B
41. F
42. E
43. D
44. C
45. G
46. A
47. H
48. E
49. H
50. G
51. B
52. C
53. A
54. D
55. F
56. C
57. G
58. E
59. D
60. A
61. C
62. F

Schedule
1. q.d. x3 weeks, 1 week off
2. q.d.
3. q.d. x3 weeks, 1 week off
4. q.d. x3 weeks, 1 week off
5. q.d.
6. Twice weekly
7. Twice weekly
8. Once weekly
9. Twice weekly
10. Twice weekly

Route of Administration
1. Transdermally
2. PO
3. Intravaginally
4. PO
5. Intravaginally
6. PO
7. Intravaginally
8. Transdermally
9. Transdermally
10. PO

Main Use/Drug Class
1. Contraception
2. Hormone Replacement
3. Hormone Replacement
4. Contraception
5. Hormone Replacement
6. Contraception
7. Hormone Replacement
8. Hormone Replacement
9. Contraception
10. Contraception

True/False
1. T
2. T
3. F
4. T
5. F
6. F
7. T
8. F
9. F
10. T

Common Strength
1. B
2. A
3. D
4. B
5. B
6. A
7. D
8. A
9. B
10. B
11. D
12. A
13. B
14. B
15. B

Multiple Choice
1. B
2. D
3. D
4. A
5. A
6. D
7. A
8. B
9. A
10. A
11. C
12. B
13. B
14. A
15. C

Sample Prescription Detrol LA
1. Tolterodine
2. Take one tablet by mouth daily
3. Three refills
4. Urinary incontinence
5. 30 days

Sample Prescription Cialis
1. Tadalafil
2. Take one tablet by mouth daily as needed
3. One refill
4. 5mg, 10mg
5. Erectile dysfunction

Sample Prescription Nuvaring
1. Etonogestrel and ethinyl estradiol
2. Insert one ring vaginally. Leave in place for three weeks, then remove for one week.
3. Five refills
4. Contraception

CHAPTER 12

Site of use
1. Ear
2. Eye
3. Eye

True/False
1. F
2. T
3. T

Matching
1. F
2. D
3. E
4. B
5. H
6. G
7. A
8. C
9. B
10. C
11. G
12. E
13. H
14. F
15. A
16. D
17. D
18. G
19. C
20. H
21. A
22. B
23. E
24. F
25. F
26. H
27. A
28. D
29. G
30. B
31. C
32. D
33. B
34. C
35. G
36. H
37. A
38. D
39. E
40. F
41. B
42. G
43. H
44. A
45. D
46. F
47. C
48. E
49. C
50. E
51. B
52. D
53. G
54. A
55. F
56. H

Frequency of Administration
1. q.i.d.
2. b.i.d.
3. q.i.d.
4. t.i.d.
5. q.i.d.
6. q.d.
7. b.i.d.
8. b.i.d.
9. q.d.
10. t.i.d.
11. b.i.d.
12. q.d.
13. t.i.d.
14. q.i.d.
15. q.d.

Correct Site of Administration
1. Eye
2. Ear
3. Eye
4. Eye
5. Ear
6. Mouth
7. Eye
8. Nose
9. Eye
10. Mouth
11. Eye
12. Eye
13. Ear
14. Nose
15. Eye
16. Ear
17. Eye
18. Eye
19. Nose
20. Eye

Main Use/Drug Class
1. Allergies
2. Glaucoma
3. Infection
4. Allergies
5. Infection
6. Glaucoma
7. Allergies
8. Infection
9. Glaucoma
10. Glaucoma
11. Glaucoma
12. Infection
13. Infection
14. Glaucoma
15. Infection

True/False
1. F
2. T
3. F
4. F
5. F
6. T
7. F
8. T
9. T
10. T

Multiple Choice
1. C
2. B
3. D
4. C
5. A
6. D
7. C
8. C
9. A
10. A
11. C
12. D
13. C
14. A
15. A

Sample Prescription Xalatan
1. Latanoprost
2. Instill one drop in both eyes every night at bedtime
3. One refill
4. 37.5 drops
5. C

Sample Prescription Cipro HC Otic
1. Ciprofloxacin and hydrocortisone
2. Instill three drops in the left ear twice daily for seven days
3. No refills
4. Ear infection
5. 150 drops
6. 25 days

Sample Prescription Abreva
1. Docosanol
2. Apply to the affected area five times daily
3. No refills
4. Cold sores

CHAPTER 13

Bacterial/Fungal
1. Fungal
2. Fungal
3. Bacterial
4. Fungal

True/False
1. T
2. T
3. T

Matching
1. F
2. A
3. E
4. D
5. H
6. B
7. C
8. G
9. A
10. C
11. B
12. G
13. E
14. D
15. F
16. H
17. G
18. D
19. A
20. H
21. C
22. E
23. F
24. B
25. F
26. H
27. A
28. C
29. E
30. G
31. B
32. D
33. F
34. D
35. B
36. A
37. C
38. E

Frequency of Administration
1. b.i.d.
2. b.i.d.
3. p.r.n.
4. t.i.d.
5. q.d.
6. b.i.d.
7. q.d.
8. b.i.d.
9. b.i.d.
10. q.d.

Main Use/Drug Class
1. Lice
2. Fungal infections
3. Acne
4. Acne
5. Lice
6. Acne
7. Lice
8. Fungal infections
9. Acne
10. Acne
11. Skin irritations
12. Acne
13. Skin irritations
14. Skin irritations
15. Acne
16. Acne
17. Acne
18. Skin irritations
19. Skin irritations
20. Acne

True/False
1. F
2. T
3. T
4. T
5. T
6. F
7. T
8. T
9. F
10. T

Multiple Choice
1. A
2. C
3. C
4. C
5. D
6. B
7. B
8. D
9. D
10. A

Sample Prescription Silvadene
1. Silver sulfadiazine
2. Apply to the affected area twice daily
3. Eight refills
4. 50g
5. Prevent and treat infections due to burns

Sample Prescription Medrol

1. Methylprednisolone
2. Use as directed
3. No refills
4. 2mg, 4mg, 8mg, 16mg, 32mg
5. Treat inflammation

Sample Prescription Zovirax

1. Acyclovir
2. Apply to cold sores fives times daily for four days
3. One refill
4. Treat cold sores

CHAPTER 14

True/False

1. T
2. T
3. T
4. F
5. T

Matching

1. C
2. H
3. D
4. F
5. E
6. G
7. A
8. B
9. C
10. E
11. H
12. F
13. A
14. D
15. B
16. G
17. C
18. H
19. E
20. A
21. F
22. G
23. D
24. B
25. D
26. G
27. C
28. E
29. B
30. A
31. F
32. H

33. C
34. G
35. B
36. F
37. A
38. D
39. E
40. H
41. G
42. C
43. F
44. A
45. B
46. D
47. H
48. E
49. D
50. H
51. A
52. C
53. B
54. F
55. E
56. G

Frequency of Administration

1. q.d.
2. q.week
3. q.d.
4. p.r.n.
5. q.d.

Parenteral/Oral/Both

1. Both
2. Both
3. Parenteral
4. Oral
5. Parenteral
6. Parenteral
7. Parenteral
8. Both
9. Oral
10. Parenteral

Main Use/Drug Class

1. Cancer
2. Cancer
3. Anemia
4. Cancer
5. Anemia
6. Anemia
7. Cancer
8. Cancer
9. Anemia
10. Anemia
11. Cancer
12. Cancer
13. Anemia
14. Anemia

15. Cancer

True/False

1. T
2. F
3. F
4. T
5. T
6. F
7. F
8. T
9. T
10. F

Multiple Choice

1. D
2. A
3. A
4. A
5. A
6. C
7. A
8. A
9. D
10. D
11. B
12. A

Sample Prescription Aromasin

1. Exemestane
2. Take one tablet by mouth daily
3. No refills
4. Cancer

Sample Prescription Cyanocobalmin

1. Vitamin B_{12}
2. Take one tablet by mouth daily
3. No refills
4. To treat or prevent vitamin B_{12} anemia
5.

CHAPTER 15

Matching

1. F
2. C
3. G
4. H
5. D
6. E
7. B
8. A
9. B
10. G
11. C
12. A

13. F
14. E
15. D

Abbreviation Matching

1. E
2. H
3. G
4. B
5. F
6. A
7. C
8. D
9. E
10. F
11. A
12. H
13. B
14. G
15. D
16. C

Frequency of Administration

1. b.i.d.
2. Infusion
3. Infusion
4. b.i.d.
5. q.d.
6. b.i.d.
7. Infusion
8. q.d.
9. b.i.d.
10. Infusion

Parenteral/Oral/Both

1. Both
2. Parenteral
3. Oral
4. Both
5. Oral
6. Parenteral
7. Parenteral
8. Both
9. Parenteral
10. Parenteral

Main Use/Drug Class

1. Organ rejection
2. Imaging
3. Organ rejection
4. Organ rejection
5. Imaging
6. Imaging
7. Organ rejection
8. Organ rejection
9. Imaging
10. Imaging

True/False

1. F
2. F
3. T
4. T
5. T
6. F
7. T
8. F
9. T
10. T

Common Strength

1. D
2. A
3. A
4. C
5. A
6. A

Multiple Choice

1. C
2. A
3. B
4. A
5. D
6. B
7. A
8. A
9. C
10. A

Sample Prescription Prograf

1. Tacrolimus
2. Take two tablets by mouth every 12 hours
3. Three refills
4. 0.5mg, 1mg, 5mg
5. Prevent organ rejection

Sample Prescription Rogaine

1. Minoxidil
2. Apply as directed twice daily
3. No refills
4. Hair growth

Glossary

A

Acne a skin condition characterized by scaly red skin, blackheads and whiteheads, pimples, and sometimes inflammation

Acquired immune deficiency syndrome (AIDS) a disease of the human immune system that makes the individual highly vulnerable to life-threatening diseases

Agonists drugs that produce the desired effects when they interact with receptors

Alimentary canal another term for the gastrointestinal tract or organs through which food travels as part of digestion

Allergy a physical response to a substance, situation, or physical state that is exaggerated compared with what the average person experiences

Alpha-blocker a drug that combines with alpha-receptors and blocks the activity of alpha receptors

Anabolic steroids hormones that are derivatives of testosterone

Analgesic an agent that relieves pain

Anaphylactic shock a severe, life-threatening hypersensitivity reaction; immediate emergency medical attention is necessary

Anatomy the scientific study of the structure of living things

Anemia a condition in which the blood does not carry enough oxygen to body tissues

Angina a disease marked by attacks of intense chest pain.

Angiotensin a protein that causes vasoconstriction

Angiotensin II the active form of angiotensin

Angiotensin II receptor blocker (ARB) a drug that blocks the vasoconstriction caused by angiotensin II

Angiotensin converting enzyme (ACE) an enzyme that converts angiotensin I to the active form angiotensin II

Antagonists drugs that block the effects of chemicals that would otherwise produce an effect through interaction with receptors

Antibacterial a substance able to inhibit or kill bacteria

Antibiotic a substance able to inhibit or kill a micro-organism

Anticoagulant a drug that hinders coagulation of the blood

Antifungal a substance able to inhibit or kill a fungus

Antihypertensive a drug that is used to treat high blood pressure

Antimicrobial a substance able to inhibit or kill a micro-organism

Antimuscarinic effects associated with slowed heart rate, increased secretion by some glands, and increased activity of certain muscles, including those of the small intestine and bladder

Antiviral a substance able to inhibit or kill a virus

Aplastic anemia a condition in which the bone marrow does not produce enough blood cells

Arrhythmia a condition in which the heartbeat is altered

Arteries blood vessels that carry blood rich in nutrients and oxygen away from the heart and throughout the body

Arthritis a condition associated with inflammation and damage to the joints of the body

Asthma a chronic lung disorder characterized by episodes of obstructed breathing

Atherosclerosis condition caused by a buildup of fatty materials such as cholesterol in the walls of arteries, causing the artery walls to thicken

Athlete's foot a common fungal infection of the skin

Autonomic nervous system (ANS) part of the peripheral nervous system associated with maintaining homeostasis

B

Bacteria single-celled microorganisms that are often aggregated into colonies and may be pathogenic

345

Bad cholesterol a lipoprotein in the blood that is associated with increased likelihood of developing atherosclerosis (low-density lipoprotein, LDL)

Behind-the-counter (BTC) drugs drugs that can be purchased without a prescription but require documentation by the pharmacist

Benign tumor a mild type of abnormal new tissue growth that has no physiologic function that does not threaten health

Beta-blocker a drug that combines with beta-receptors to block the activity of a beta-receptor, decreasing the heart rate and forcing contractions of the heart

Bile a fluid produced by the liver and passed into the digestive system that aids with digestion and the processing of cholesterol and other fats

Bile acid resin medications that bind with certain components of bile in the gastrointestinal tract and can aid in lowering cholesterol

Blood vessels closed system of tubes in the body that circulate blood

Bone an organ of the skeleton

Brain the portion of the central nervous system contained within the skull

Brand name a unique, proprietary name selected by a pharmaceutical company that produces the drug

Bronchodilator a device or medication that expands or dilates the airways

Bronchospasm a muscle contraction of the airway muscles that constricts breathing

C

Calcium channel blocker (CCB) drugs that block calcium channels in the muscle cells of the heart and blood vessels to prevent calcium from entering these cells, resulting in reduced blood pressure

Cancer a malignant tumor that has unlimited potential for growth

Carcinogenicity drug effects that cause cancer

Cardiovascular a term relating to the heart and blood vessels

Cardiovascular system the organ system that distributes blood throughout the body

Cartilage elastic tissue of the skeleton

Central nervous system (CNS) the brain and spinal cord

Chemotherapy a term used for the treatment of cancer with medications

Chronic obstructive pulmonary disease (COPD) a form of lung disease characterized by airway narrowing or obstruction and a slower rate of breathing

Clotting factors proteins in the blood that work with platelets to produce blood clots

Complementary and alternative medicine (CAM) therapies outside of evidence-based medicine

Congestive heart failure a condition in which the heart is unable to maintain adequate circulation of blood in the body

Controlled substances drugs that are regulated by the Drug Enforcement Agency because of their potential for abuse

Cranial nerves nerves in the peripheral nervous system that originate in the brain

D

Dermatologic pertaining to the skin and its structure, functions, and diseases

Desiccated thyroid thyroid glands that have been dried and powdered for therapeutic use

Diabetes a chronic condition associated with how the body processes sugar that can be life-threatening

Digestion the process of breaking down food into simpler chemicals

Diuretic a drug that increases urination and lowers blood pressure

Drug Enforcement Agency (DEA) the federal agency that regulates controlled substances

Drug interaction effects that may result when a patient takes two drugs simultaneously

Drugs substances intended for use in the diagnosis, cure, mitigation, treatment, or prevention of disease

E

Erectile dysfunction (ED) condition in males associated with a failure to have or maintain an erection (impotence)

Erythrocytes red blood cells (RBCs)

Esophagus passage for food to travel to the stomach

Estrogen hormone associated with the female reproductive system

Evidence-based medicine prescribing medications for clinical use on the basis of scientific data

Expectorate to spit out

F

Food and Drug Administration (FDA) the federal agency that approves drugs for sale in the United States

Fungus a type of organism that was formerly classified as a plant without chlorophyll and includes molds, rusts, mushrooms, and yeasts

G

Gallbladder accessory organ associated with the process of digestion

Gastrointestinal referring to digestive activities (e.g., stomach, intestines)

Gastrointestinal tract the system of organs through which food travels during digestion

Generic name a specific, nonproprietary name assigned to a drug by the United States Adopted Names (USAN) Council

Good cholesterol a lipoprotein in the blood that is associated with decreased likelihood of developing atherosclerosis (high-density lipoprotein, HDL)

Gross anatomy the study of structures within the body that are large enough to be seen by the naked eye

H

Hematological effects drug effects that alter the composition of the blood

Hematology the study of blood, the blood-forming organs, and blood diseases

Hemophilia one type of bleeding disorder in which the blood does not clot normally because of clotting factor deficiency

Hemostatic agents medications that slow some types of bleeding by slowing the rate of the breakdown of blood clots

Hepatotoxicity drug effects that damage the liver

Homeostasis the ability of the body to maintain stable internal physiological balance, such as body temperature and the pH of blood, when environmental conditions change

Hormones chemicals in the body that are secreted by glands into the bloodstream and function to regulate other processes in the body

Human immunodeficiency virus (HIV) the virus that causes AIDS

Hyperlipidemia a condition of excess lipids in the blood

Hypersensitivity an allergic reaction

Hypertension abnormally high blood pressure

Hyperthyroidism a condition in which the thyroid gland produces too much of the thyroid hormones

Hypothyroidism a condition in which the thyroid gland produces too little of the thyroid hormones

I

Imaging agents medications that are administered to improve the visibility of body structures for imaging diagnostic tests, such as X-rays and CT scans

Immunization the process of administering a vaccine to protect against a disease (this term is often used interchangeably with the term *vaccination*)

Immunobiologic an agent associated with the physiological reactions of the immune system

Immunology the study of the immune system especially related to health and disease

Impetigo a contagious bacterial infection of the skin

Impotence a condition in males associated with a failure to have or maintain an erection (erectile dysfunction)

Inactivated vaccine a killed vaccine that is given by injection into the muscle

Inhalation the process by which air or medication is taken into the lungs

Inhaler a device used to deliver medication to the lungs via inhalation

Insulin a hormone produced by the pancreas that regulates blood sugar levels.

Integumentary system system containing the skin, hair, and nails

Intramuscular (IM) drug is injected into a muscle

Intravenous (IV) drug is injected directly into a vein

J

Jock itch a common fungal infection of the skin

Joint point of contact between bones or cartilage

K

Keratoses crusty or scaly patches of skin

L

Leukocytes white blood cells (WBCs)

Lipid non-water-soluble substances such as fats that are important in the body

Lipoprotein proteins that conjugate with lipids

Live, attenuated vaccine a weakened influenza vaccine that is sprayed into the nostrils

Liver accessory organ associated with the process of digestion

M

Malignant tumor an abnormal new growth of tissue that has no physiologic function; malignant tumors usually threaten health and can lead to death

Menopause time when the natural cessation of menstruation occurs in women

Metastasis a term to describe the spread of cancer to one or more other parts of the body

Metered-dose inhaler (MDI) an often pocket-sized device that delivers a fixed dose of medication upon each use

Microscopic anatomy the study of structures within the body that can be seen only with microscopes

N

Narcotic a drug derived from the opium plant that changes the way the body senses pain and thereby provides relief from pain

National Drug Code (NDC) a specific set of numbers assigned to a drug by the pharmaceutical company that produces it

Nebulizer a device that converts a liquid solution into a fine mist to deliver medication to the lungs via inhalation

Nephrotoxicity drug effects that damage the kidneys

Nerve impulses transmission of sensations along nerves

Neuron nerve cell

O

Ocular pertaining to the eye

Oncology the study of cancer

Ophthalmic pertaining to the eye

Oral contraceptives medications that usually contain a combination of a progestin and an estrogen, but sometimes only a progestin, that prevent pregnancy

Osteoporosis a condition in which bones become brittle, characterized by decreased bone mass and decreased bone density

Otic pertaining to the ear

Ovaries Female reproductive glands

Over-the-counter (OTC) drugs drugs that can be purchased without a prescription

P

Pancreas accessory organ associated with the process of digestion

Parenteral route of administration other than the digestive system

Partial agonists drugs that produce only partial effects through receptor interactions

Pathogenic capable of causing disease

Pathophysiology the study of abnormal body functions that can be caused by diseases or other processes that are not normal

Peripheral nervous system (PNS) nerves outside of the central nervous system

Pharmacokinetics the study of the absorption, distribution, metabolism, and excretion of drugs in the body after they are administered.

Pharmacology the study of how drugs or other chemicals work in the body

Physiology the study of the functions within living things

Plasma the liquid component of blood, which consists of water, nutrients, hormones, salts, proteins, and waste products

Platelets a type of blood cell made in the bone marrow that plays an important role in blood clotting (also known as thrombocytes)

Pneumonia one type of lung infection that can be treated with anti-infective medications

Poison Prevention Packaging Act (PPPA) federal law that requires child-resistant closures on most prescription and nonprescription medications

Progestin hormone associated with the female reproductive system

Protein naturally occurring complex substances that include many essential biological compounds such as enzymes, hormones, and antibodies

R

Receptors minute specialized surfaces in various parts of the body that provide the sites of action for medications

Respiratory referring to the lungs and other breathing passages

Respiratory syncytial virus (RSV) A virus that causes serious lower respiratory tract infections in children and infants

Ringworm a common fungal infection of the skin

Route of administration the way a drug is administered

S

Salivary glands accessory organ associated with the process of digestion

Side effects unintended effects caused by a drug

Skeletal muscle one of three types of muscle in the body that is commonly attached to bones

Skeleton a collection of bones that provides structure and protection

Spinal cord portion of the central nervous system that extends from the brain

Spinal nerves nerves in the peripheral nervous system that originate from the spinal cord

Subcutaneous (SC, SQ) drug that is injected into the fatty tissue just below the skin (note that the abbreviation for subcutaneous can be the source of medication errors)

Sulfa drug a type of antibiotic

T

Teratogenicity drug effects that disrupt normal fetal development

Testes male reproductive glands

Testosterone hormone associated with the male reproductive system

Third party prescription coverage through a patient's health care insurance

Thrombocytes a type of blood cell made in the bone marrow that plays an important role in blood clotting (also known as platelets)

Thrombolytic a drug that breaks down blood clots

Transplant rejection the body's attack of a transplanted organ by the immune system of the person who receives the organ

Tumor an abnormal new growth of tissue that possesses no physiological function

U

United States Adopted Names (USAN) Council group sponsored by the American Medical Association (AMA), United States Pharmacopeial Convention (USPC), and the American Pharmacists Association (APhA) that assigns generic names to drugs; the council determines generic names for drugs using special syllables called "stems," which can then be grouped by therapeutic class or category

V

Vaccination the process of administering a vaccine to protect against a disease (this term is often used interchangeably with the term *immunization*)

Vaccine a preparation of microorganisms that have been treated to make them harmless and is administered to produce immunity to a disease

Vasodilator a drug that causes blood vessels to dilate

Veins blood vessels that carry blood toward the heart

Virus any of a large group of submicroscopic agents that can cause infection

W

Wheeze to breathe with difficulty, often accompanied by a whistling sound